A Colour Guide to Holistic Oral Care

A Practical Approach

Janet Griffiths

Senior Dental Officer
Cardiff Dental Hospital and School
Cardiff, UK

Steve Boyle

Dental Services Manager
Gwent Community Trust
Gwent, UK

Copyright © 1993 Mosby–Year Book Europe
Printed by BPCC Hazell Books Ltd, Aylesbury, England
ISBN 0 7234 1779 2

All rights reserved. No reproduction, copy or transmission of this publication may be made without written permission.

No part of this publication may be reproduced, copied or transmitted save with written permission or in accordance with the provisions of the Copyright Act 1956 (as amended), or under the terms of any licence permitting limited copying issued by the Copyright Licensing Agency, 33–34 Alfred Place, London, WC1E 7DP.

Any person who does any unauthorised act in relation to this publication may be liable to criminal prosecution and civil claims for damages.

A CIP catalogue record for this book is available from the British Library.

For full details of all Mosby titles please write to Mosby–Year Book Europe, Lynton House, 7–12 Tavistock Square, London WC1H 9LB, England.

Contents

Preface	iv
Acknowledgements	v
Dedication	vi
Introduction: How to Use This Guide	1

Section 1 Practical Oral Care 5
1 Oral Health and Disease 6
2 Basic Principles and Practice of Oral Care 23
3 Child Dental Health 42
4 Oral Care for Older People 56
5 Dental Services and the Dental Team 71

Section 2 A Guide to Oral Assessment with Colour Photographs 85
6 Oral Assessment 87
7 Role of the Nurse Manager in Promoting Oral Care 99
8 Oral Effects of Medication 107
9 Aids to Oral Self-Care, Rehabilitation and Independence 112
Colour Plates *Between pages 106 and 107*

Section 3 At-Risk Groups: People with a Special Need 127
10 Physical Disability and Sensory Impairment 131
11 People with Learning Disabilities 151
12 People Suffering from Mental Illness 162
13 Medically Compromised Patients 182
14 Oral Infections and Related Conditions 194
15 Malignant Disease and its Treatment 205
16 Oral Care of the Dysphagic, Dependent and Terminally Ill 217

Section 4 Oral Health Promotion: Approaches and Practices 225
17 Approaches to Oral Health Promotion 228
18 Practical Oral Health Promotion 241

Appendix 1: Resource Addresses	249
Appendix 2: Disabled Living Centres	251
Further Reading	255
Glossary	256
Index	259

Preface

This guide is primarily written for nurses, other health care professionals and all carers who are involved in some way in assisting or providing oral care for people. We have designed it to be used in a practical way and, hopefully, we have provided some guidance and direction for most situations.

We have both been involved in providing primary and secondary dental care in many scenarios over the years, and between us we have experience in delivering dental care in hospitals, general dental practices, and community dental services throughout the UK and in developing countries. Much of that dental care has been for people with special needs, i.e. people who are not completely self caring and who require varying degrees of support to meet their daily oral needs.

As part of our roles we have both been called upon many times to provide teaching and/or education in oral care and we have always encountered the lack of a suitable back-up text. We hope this guide will go some way to meeting this deficiency! We have endeavoured to provide accurate, practical information in an accessible form.

It is also intended that this book be used in a practical way and rather than read it in a conventional sense, we would like you to consult first the 'How to use this guide' introduction.

All health care professionals are now aware of the global strategy of 'Health For All, 2000'. One of its strongest tenets is for all members of the health care team to work together. We hope that by empowering the health professional and the carer with the skills and knowledge for effective oral care, we have contributed in some small way to that aim.

Please do write to us with your views and suggestions for any sections of care we may have missed.

Janet Griffiths
Steve Boyle

Acknowledgements

This guide would not have been possible without the support of many people. In addition to the acknowledgements in the text, we would like to express our thanks to colleagues in the dental and other professions for their advice, support and constructive criticism in preparing this text, especially Teresa Goss, Sue Greening, Liz Hunt, Bruce Hunter, and Josie Prior.

The manual would be incomplete without the colour section and illustrations. We are particularly grateful to colleagues who have allowed us to reproduce their slides. Our thanks go to Richard Green, Mike Harrison, Shelagh Thompson and to the Dental Illustration Department, Cardiff Dental Hospital, for allowing us to raid their slide resources. We are indebted to Frank Hartles, head of the Dental Illustration Department, and in particular to Edwina Wyver for the excellent line drawings and illustrations. We would also like to thank our secretaries, Sue and Debbie, for all their help.

Finally, grateful thanks also go to our respective partners, Brad and Shelagh, for their patient support during the long and antisocial hours we spent at the word processor.

JEG and SB

Dedication

To the residents of the Royal Earlswood Hospital, Surrey and the Greaves Hall Hospital, Merseyside, and to the people of Beira, Mozambique, who gave us our earliest professional experiences of 'special needs'; and to the many people with disabilities and their 'carers' who inspired us to write this guide.

Introduction: How to Use This Guide

Section 1: Practical Oral Care

This section of the guide forms the core knowledge and skills required by all health professionals and carers undertaking oral care. Many of the later, more specialised chapters refer back to this section, and so if you only read one section, this is the one to concentrate on!

A description of the main oral diseases is followed by the basic principles and practice of oral care that a self-caring adult would be expected to carry out. For people in your care, this is the level of care at which you should be aiming to achieve oral health.

The two broad groups of children and of older people and their differing oral needs are then examined.

The section concludes with a chapter on dental services and the dental team. This chapter has been included in this section to enable the health professional to access effectively the most appropriate aspect of the service. For the reader outside the UK there will be differences in the organisation of dental services.

After reading Section 1, look at the most appropriate section for your clients' needs. Most health care professionals will require criteria for assessing oral health needs.

Section 2: A Guide to Oral Assessment

Section 2 is aimed particularly at the nurse providing care in a hospital or community setting. The guidelines, criteria and procedures are based on a wide variety of settings, and this section should be used as a check list for the requirements for an environment which is supportive of oral health, rather than the converse which often creates barriers to oral health.

The first chapter examines key indicators for oral health and reviews current assessment systems. It is intended that this will assist in the nursing process and the formulation of care plans based on meeting an individual's oral needs.

The suggested role of the nurse manager is then outlined in the following chapter as the key individual controlling resources and staff. Although identified as a nurse manager, this key person may have a variety of roles. However, the principle underpinning this chapter is that one person should oversee the development of oral care, keep it on the agenda, facilitate training and manage the required resources.

Chapter 8 summarises the major oral side-effects of drugs and medications and their effects on oral health. Later sections provide more detail on the specific oral side-effects of medications.

The section closes with a detailed review of the tools and equipment needed to provide oral care. It is recognised that many clients will require varying degrees of assistance to meet their oral needs.

Now select the chapter most appropriate to your client group for an overview of their oral condition, the effects on oral health, and how oral care should be modified.

Section 3: At-Risk Groups: People with a Special Need

This section provides a comprehensive review of most disabling conditions and diseases and their effects on oral health, including the effects of medication and treatment.

It is inevitable that there will be an overlap between chapters in this section due to the multifactorial nature of illness and the overlap between conditions. The authors have grouped the conditions in the following order after consultation with specialists and, where appropriate, people with the conditions:

- Physical disability.
- Learning disability.
- Mental illness.
- Medically compromised patients.
- Infectious diseases.
- Malignant diseases.
- Dysphagic, dependant and terminally ill patients.

Although there will be inevitable exclusions and oversights, about which the authors would welcome comments, we believe that we have covered most modifying factors, from the perspective of oral health, via this approach.

Section 4: Oral Health Promotion: Approaches and Practices

This section is designed to address the health promotion aspect of oral health care. This is a central theme of primary health care, with almost everyone being familiar with the maxim 'prevention is better than cure'. This section examines how oral health promotion can be more fully integrated into general health promotion. There is no reason why the mouth should be separated from the rest of the body!

In Chapter 17, a widely accepted model of health promotion is used as a method of demonstrating how oral health can be considered within general health promotion. Although at first it may appear that this section is aimed at the specialised group of health care workers with clearly identified roles in health promotion, we recognise that health promotion should form a part of every health intervention. Even for the most dependent individual there is always some potential for health promotion and some way of maximising the potential for self-care.

Chapter 18 provides clear practical guidance for health promotion throughout life. This is to enable the health care professional to be alert to oral health issues and to use this awareness to promote oral health.

Finally, we hope that you will use this guide as part of your daily health care activities. It was not produced for a 'read-once-and-onto-the-shelf' approach!

Section 1

Practical Oral Care

This section forms the central core knowledge that is required by all health professionals and carers involved in holistic health care. The basic preventive methods of the commonest oral diseases and methods for maintaining oral health are described in Chapters 1 and 2. These two chapters are concerned with the 'self-caring adult' and the principles of oral care they would follow. The differing needs of children and older age are examined in Chapters 3 and 4. The section concludes with a detailed examination of dental services and the dental team in the United Kingdom. This is to assist the health professional or carer to help those in their care to access the most appropriate service and member of the dental team.

1 Oral Health and Disease

1.1 Oral Disease
1.2 Periodontal Disease
1.3 Chronic Inflammatory Periodontal Disease
   Causes and modifying factors
   Prevention
   Summary of preventive methods
1.4 Dental Caries
   Signs and symptoms of dental caries
   Cause of dental caries
   Factors affecting dental decay
   The role of toothbrushing in preventing dental decay
   Other methods of plaque control
   Summary of preventive methods for dental caries
1.5 Role of Saliva in Oral Health
1.6 Oral Cancer
   Risk factors for oral cancer
1.7 Distribution of Oral Disease
   Dental caries
   Periodontal disease
   Tooth loss
1.8 General Disability and Oral Handicap
1.9 Phases in Prevention of Oral Disease and Oral Ill Health
   Primary prevention
   Secondary prevention
   Tertiary prevention
1.10 Summary
1.11 References

1.1 Oral Disease

The 'World's Commonest Disease'[1] is actually composed of two common diseases – periodontal (gum) disease and dental caries (tooth decay) – and is largely self-inflicted. As the mouth acts as a 'mirror' of general health, there may also be oral manifestations of general diseases and conditions. In addition, there are the rarer oral infections and the more life-threatening oral cancers.

1.2 Periodontal Disease

Although periodontal disease is the single largest cause of tooth loss in adults[2], the early signs and symptoms of periodontal disease, which are gums that bleed when brushing, are often not recognised as abnormal (*Colour Plate* 3). Other later signs of periodontal disease, such as receding gums and loose teeth, are still often seen as part of the ageing process by many people (*Colour Plate* 4). Although 95% of the adult population will exhibit some effects of periodontal disease, the severity of disease varies enormously, and it poses a higher threat to the dentition of approximately 10–15% of the population who are more susceptible to the damaging effects.[3]

Periodontal disease is a collective term for a number of conditions which affect the supporting fibres linking the teeth to the surrounding bone and the associated tissues covering them. *Figure 1.1* shows a diagrammatic cross-section of a healthy tooth.

In lay terms, the 'gum' is a description of all the mucous membranes that cover the supporting bones and musculature of the jaws. In anatomical terms, there is a differentiation between the 'gingival tissue' which consists of free and attached tissue over the bone in which are inserted the roots of the teeth, and the rest of the soft tissues in the mouth.

1.3 Chronic Inflammatory Periodontal Disease

The commonest of the periodontal diseases is chronic inflammatory periodontal disease. This condition often begins in childhood with inflamed gum margins. The reddened, swollen gum margins bleed when brushed as they are more fragile than healthy gum tissue. This stage is referred to as 'gingivitis' and is usually controllable with more effective toothbrushing (*Colour Plate* 3). The condition is reversible and no lasting damage to the gums should occur. However, the condition can progress to 'chronic periodontitis' in which the fibres and bone supporting the teeth are affected (*Colour Plate* 4). This may progress to loosening of the teeth and infections which result in the tooth requiring extraction. Although virtually all adults exhibit some effects of chronic periodontitis, the rate at which the condition progresses varies enormously between individuals.

Causes and modifying factors

Periodontal disease is caused by 'dental plaque'. This is a descriptive term for the layer of bacteria on teeth which is present in all mouths. Plaque will build up on any surface in the mouth, whether natural or artificial, but only to any appreciable degree in those areas where it is not removed by the normal movements of speech and eating.

The normal anatomy of the teeth and gums creates a space in which plaque can accumulate, and a number of other factors can contribute to a potentially damaging build-up. These factors include crooked teeth, badly adapted fillings and some types of dentures. In some parts of the mouth, the formation of 'calculus' or 'tartar' will act as a rough surface on teeth, so permitting a greater build-up of plaque (*Colour Plates* **4, 5, 6**).

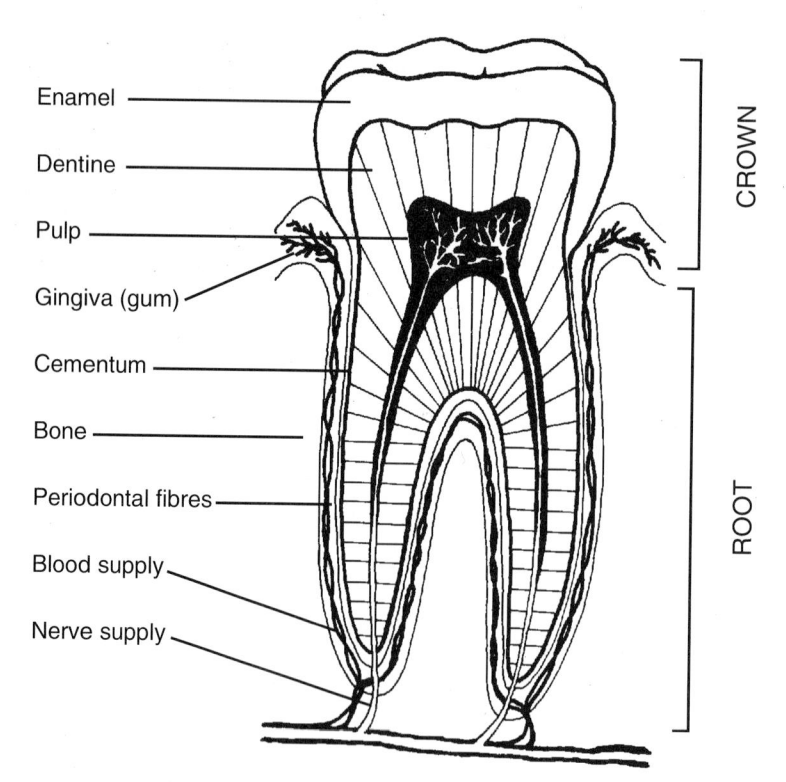

Figure 1.1 Diagrammatic cross-section of a healthy molar tooth.

After a period of several days the colony of micro-organisms in the plaque will produce enough toxins and by-products to initiate a response from the body. This is the normal inflammatory response to any injury or infection. If the irritant plaque is not removed, this response becomes chronic and progressive and there is some tissue destruction and repair. Eventually the supporting bone and periodontal fibres are destroyed and replaced by fibrous tissue.

There are variations in the bacterial composition of dental plaque between individuals and even between different sites in the mouth. This may account for some of the differences seen in the rate at which disease progresses. Hormonal and metabolic changes during pregnancy and puberty, or linked to disorders such as diabetes, can also alter the response, but in many cases there is no identifiable reason. As in all chronic infections, the response of the individual's immune system will alter the progress of the disease and there is no reason to suggest that chronic periodontal disease should be an exception. Any chronic debilitating condition can affect the gums either directly or by impairing the individual's ability to maintain effective oral hygiene.

Prevention

The main approach to prevention is to control the formation of plaque. Even though it is not feasible to sterilise the mouth and rid it permanently of bacteria, plaque can be prevented from accumulating at sites in the mouth and reaching the stage of provoking an inflammatory condition. Plaque control depends on the individual being able to maintain effective oral hygiene. One of the main aims of this guide is to enable individuals who are dependent to some extent on others for their daily needs to achieve this.

Summary of preventive methods

Chapter 2 describes the basic principles of plaque control for the self-caring adult. These consist of:

- Daily removal of plaque from the gum margins.
- Regular removal of calculus (tartar) by dental professionals.
- Regular dental attendance.

1.4 Dental Caries

The main condition affecting the tooth itself is dental caries or dental decay (*Colour Plates* **7, 8, 9**). Dental caries starts in the outer covering of enamel with a small area losing some of its mineral content. Once the enamel is breached, the process continues through the softer layer of dentine underneath. This can undermine the structure of the tooth and a

Holistic Oral Care

cavity may form. The cavity, if untreated, will continue to enlarge until the living pulp is reached and direct infection will occur. The resulting infection can track the length of the root canal and an abscess may form (*Figure 1.2*). The sequence of events can be summarised by the equation:

Plaque + Sugar ⟶ Acid + Tooth Surface ⟶ Dental Caries

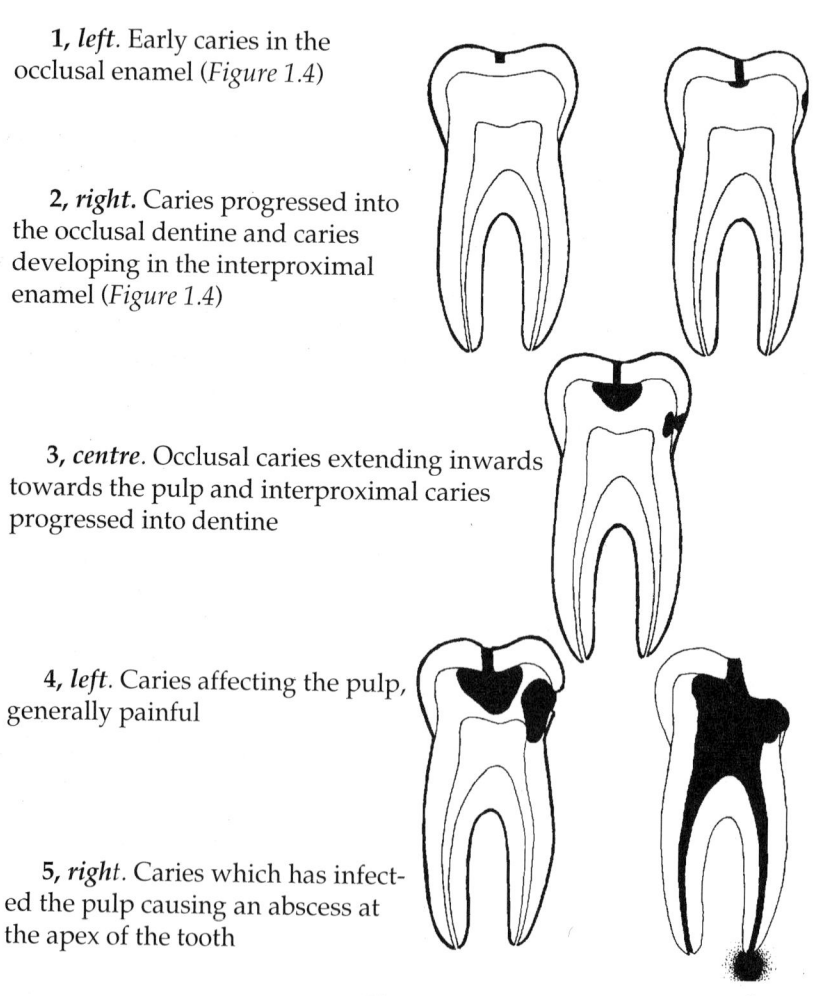

1, left. Early caries in the occlusal enamel (*Figure 1.4*)

2, right. Caries progressed into the occlusal dentine and caries developing in the interproximal enamel (*Figure 1.4*)

3, centre. Occlusal caries extending inwards towards the pulp and interproximal caries progressed into dentine

4, left. Caries affecting the pulp, generally painful

5, right. Caries which has infected the pulp causing an abscess at the apex of the tooth

Figure 1.2. The decay process

Signs and symptoms of dental caries

Healthy enamel and dentine form an effective insulation for the nerve fibres in the pulp chamber and a healthy tooth will not react to changes in temperature unless they are excessive. The sensitivity experienced by some people is often due to the transmission of temperature changes from an exposed root cementum to the nerve.

In the earlier stages of dental caries, the tooth may be painful only in the transmission of hot and cold, which is due to loss of insulating enamel and dentine. The symptoms and signs of the later stages are obvious to the individual, with severe pain and swelling as the contents of the pulp chamber become inflamed.

It may take several years for significant damage in the form of a large cavity to develop and the early stages may be completely symptom-free and painless.

Cause of dental caries

There is normally a balance at the surface of the tooth enamel between mineral built into the surface of the tooth being lost to saliva and being laid down again. This balance will be disturbed by the presence of acids, which will result in a net loss of mineral. If the mineral balance is not restored, dental caries will occur. Acid derives from the bacteria present in dental plaque, as the bacteria break down certain dietary sugars, particularly sucrose and fructose for energy and growth. As this happens the plaque colony will grow and help to retain the acid in contact with the tooth, and thus promote further demineralisation.

Factors affecting dental decay

The single largest factor in promoting dental caries is the number of times that sugars are consumed. It takes just a couple of minutes for the bacteria in plaque to produce enough acid to tip the mineral balance towards a loss of mineral. This imbalance (sometimes called an 'acid attack') takes up to an hour to neutralise. Another ingestion of sugar during that period will prolong the time during which the mouth is acidic and therefore promotes dental caries.

Saliva can help to neutralise the acids produced by plaque bacteria. There is a reduction in normal salivary flow at night; this creates even more favourable conditions for bacterial plaque to proliferate. In later chapters the effects of certain medications on saliva flow will be highlighted as leaving individuals more susceptible to dental caries.

The resistance of the tooth to dental caries appears to vary between people, although this observation is often wrongly ascribed as an explanation for why it occurs.

As the process of demineralisation, remineralisation and acid attacks is not easy to explain without a grounding in a scientific background, other explanations are sometimes used and this can result in over-simplification. Low resistance to decay is an explanation that should be used with caution as it implies that there is little that can be done by the person to control and prevent further dental caries.

Besides reducing the frequency and the quantity of sugar consumption, the other important factor in preventing dental caries is fluoride. The most important effect of fluoride is to prevent the loss of calcium and phosphate at the surface of the tooth. To be most effective it should be used on a daily basis, either in drinking water, toothpaste or in daily supplements. Chapters 2 and 3 provide more detailed information on the use of fluoride.

No other supplement, such as calcium, has been shown to have any preventive effect on teeth. Similarly, malnutrition or dietary deficiencies during pregnancy have little effect on the infant's teeth, except in very rare cases. Once calcium has been laid down in the tooth during development, only the decay process can remove it; there is no mechanism for a fetus to remove mineral during pregnancy.

The role of toothbrushing in preventing dental decay

Toothbrushing alone will not prevent dental caries. The sites in the mouth where dental caries begins are very difficult, if not impossible, to render plaque free with a toothbrush. These sites are the cracks and fissures on the chewing surfaces of the molars (occlusal surfaces) (*Colour Plate* **9**) and in between the teeth (interproximal surfaces) (*Colour Plate* **8**, *Figure 1.3*). Toothbrushing does have a vital preventive role as a method for applying fluoride toothpaste, and it is of course the main preventive tool for gum disease.

Interproximal areas

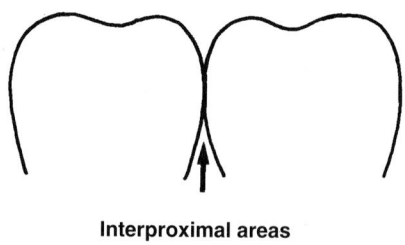

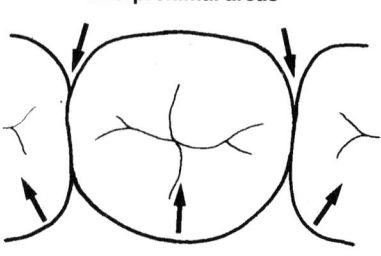

Occlusal fissures

Figure 1.3 Occlusal and proximal surfaces

Oral Health and Disease

Other methods of plaque control
While it is impossible to eliminate plaque on a practical level, and indeed not even completely necessary, there are antiseptic agents which can suppress it. For people with special needs these may be a useful aid to oral hygiene. Chapter 9 describes oral hygiene aids and their appropriate use. They are referred to throughout the guide.

Eating fibrous foods like carrots and apples does not have any demonstrable effect on plaque levels, but they are certainly preferable to sweets as healthy snacks.

Summary of preventive methods for dental caries
Chapter 2 describes in detail the methods for prevention of dental caries for the self-caring adult. These consist of:

- Reducing the consumption, particularly the number of intakes, of sugar in food and drink.
- Cleaning the teeth and gums every day with a fluoride toothpaste.
- Regular dental attendance for detection of early problems.

1.5 Role of Saliva in Oral Health

It has been increasingly demonstrated that saliva has an important role in maintaining oral health. Its functions are:

- Lubrication of the soft tissues.
- Mechanical flushing of food and debris.
- Neutralisation of acids caused by plaque and sugars.
- Providing minerals to strengthen the tooth surface.
- Anti-bacterial effect.

These properties have obvious benefits in speech, mastication and swallowing, and in maintaining the health of both hard and soft tissues. The implications of reduced salivary flow in relation to specific conditions will be dealt with in later chapters.

1.6 Oral Cancer

Oral cancer is obviously the most life-threatening of all oral diseases and accounts for 1.2% of all malignancies.[4] Although there have been changes in the numbers of cases in different parts of the mouth and oral cavity, intra-oral cancers are increasing, especially in females.

Unfortunately, many cases are only diagnosed at an advanced stage as the early stages are frequently symptom-free (*Colour Plates* **28, 29**, **30**).

Late diagnosis has adverse effects on the patient's prognosis and life expectancy. Prevention or reduction of the risk factors for oral cancers is of vital importance, as is early detection.

Risk factors for oral cancer

Depending on the site of the oral cancer, there are a number of associated risk factors:

- Sunlight.
- Tobacco.
- Alcohol.
- Dental factors.
- Nutritional deficiencies.
- Infections.
- Viruses.

Exposure to sunlight has been identified as a factor in cancer of the lip, with a higher incidence in people with outdoor occupations.[5,6] The lower incidence of lip cancer amongst women has been been attributed to the use of cosmetics[7], while the use of lip protection has produced a decrease in the number of lip cancers in the United States of America.[8]

Tobacco, whether smoked, chewed or taken as snuff, is reported to be an important factor in the aetiology of oral cancer.[9] Research has demonstrated a relationship between cigarette smoking and cancer of the mouth.[10,11] Pipe-smoking is linked with cancer of the lip which may be partly due to the excessive heat generated.[12] Reverse smoking, the practice of smoking with the lit end inside the mouth, common in some Asian countries, is linked with cancer of the hard palate.[13]

The use of snuff, and other smokeless uses of tobacco such as betel quid chewing and tobacco pouches, have also been strongly implicated as agents involved in the rise in oral cancers.[14-16] It is not clear whether tobacco has a direct effect on oral tissues or whether it makes the oral tissues more susceptible to carcinogens or cancer-producing viruses.[12]

High alcohol consumption is implicated in the aetiology of oral cancer; occupations with easy access to alcohol show a higher incidence[17] as compared with a lower incidence in religious groups who abstain.[18] The risk is significantly increased when alcohol is consumed with tobacco.[19] The rise in consumption patterns of alcohol and cigarette smoking in females is linked with the rising proportion of female cases of oral cancer.[20]

Although it seems that local factors, for example poor oral hygiene and local irritations due to poorly fitting dentures, may be risk factors, scientific confirmation is lacking.[12] Nutritional deficiencies may increase susceptibility to oral cancer as well as to certain lesions of the mucous membrane, which become infected by candidal organisms.[21] Viral infections, in particular herpes simplex and human papilloviruses[12], and fungal infections[21] are also under suspicion.

Oral Health and Disease

One of the roles for those involved in oral care is early detection of malignant and pre-malignant stages because early diagnosis is so important to the outcome of treatment. Section 2 illustrates some of the conditions which could arouse suspicion.

1.7 Distribution of Oral Disease

Dental caries
Over the centuries, there have been several changes in the rate of dental caries which have closely mirrored changing patterns of sugar consumption. *Figure 1.4* shows the dramatic increase that occurred from the 17th century onwards once imported cane sugar became more widely available. Changes in techniques for milling flour produced a more refined product which was less wearing on teeth and did not eradicate the fissures of the chewing surfaces where much decay starts. Further increases were seen due to the import of wheat products which substantially changed eating patterns.

Sugar consumption rose during the 19th century with the removal of tariffs; this rise was only temporarily halted by sugar rationing in both World Wars. These temporary declines in sugar consumption were also accompanied by temporary reductions in dental caries.

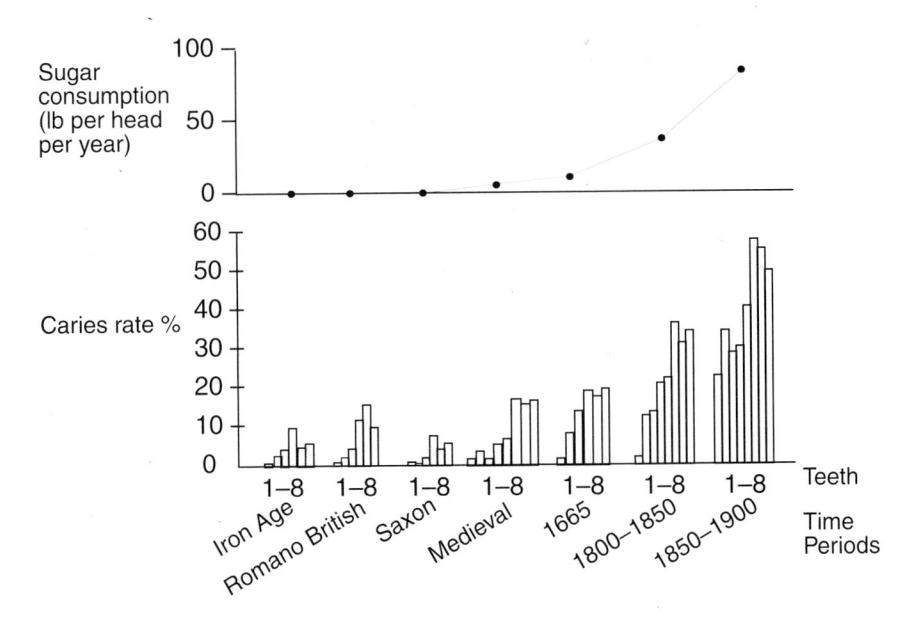

Figure 1.4 Historical sugar consumption and caries rate in the permanent dentitions of British populations. By permission of Professor C.E. Renson.[28]

Holistic Oral Care

Although sugar consumption has been fairly constant at an average 40kg per person per year for the last few decades[22], there has been a dramatic reduction in the amount of dental caries in industrialised countries. Studies from the World Health Organization (WHO) Global Data Bank have shown large decreases during the 1970s. *Figure 1.5* shows dental caries trends in 12-year-old children in nine industrialised countries. The index used, DMFT, is the number of decayed, missing and filled adult teeth.

The main reasons underlying the fall in dental caries are:

- Wider use of fluoride-containing toothpaste.
- Greater awareness of the importance of good dental health.
- Greater use of dental services.
- Increased availability of dental resources.
- A more preventive approach adopted by dentists in their use of dental health education, fissure sealants and topical fluoride.

Although the total consumption of sugar remains high, there have been changes in patterns of consumption in social and cultural groups.[23] Dental caries is very much a social class-related condition[24] and it still remains a substantial health problem. When examined in more detail, there is a demonstrable gradient *(Figure 1.6)* which shows the dental decay experienced by 12-year-old children in the UK in 1988.[25] Within districts, it has been shown that many factors associated with social deprivation are also linked with high decay rates. Apparent racial differences are mainly due to social deprivation, including language barriers.[26]

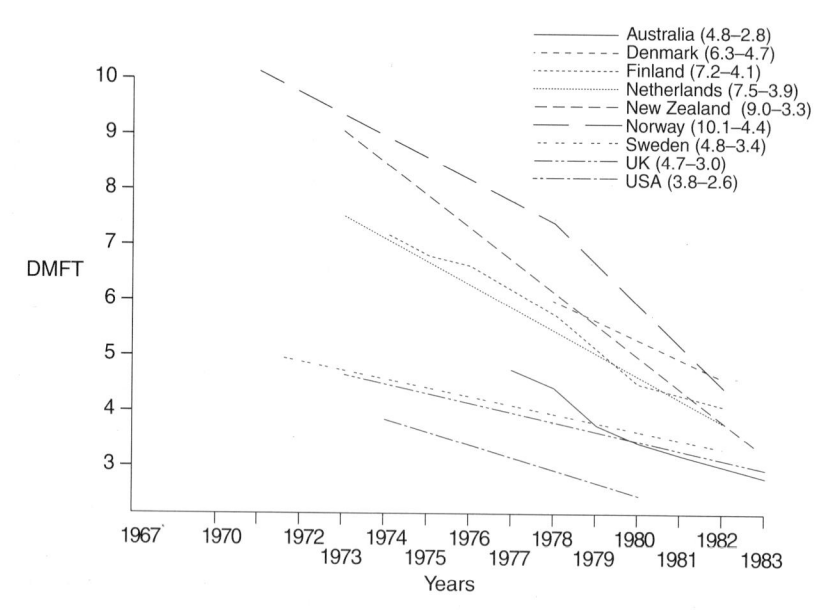

Figure 1.5 International trends in dental caries 1967–1983, DMFT at 12 years. By permission of Professor C.E. Renson.[28]

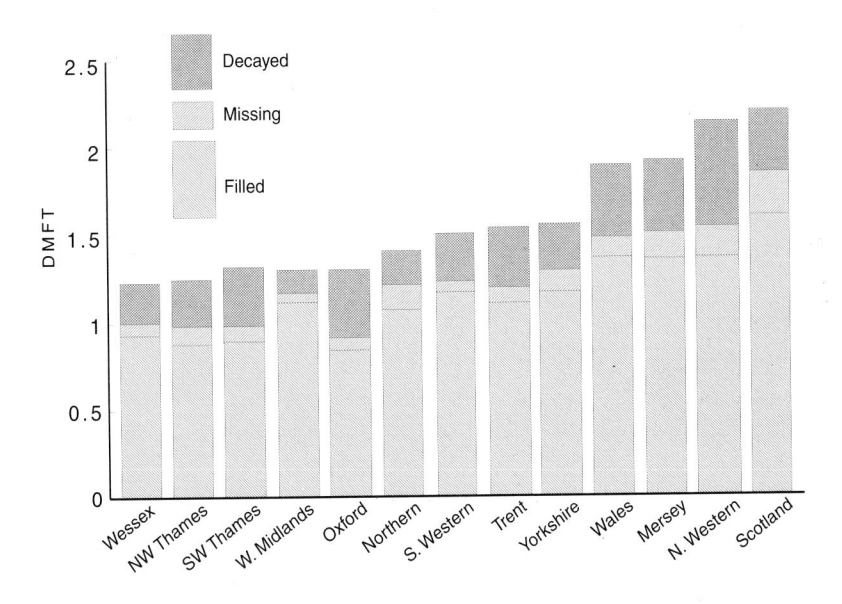

Figure 1.6 Dental decay experienced by 12-year-old children in the UK (1988–1989). By permission of Macmillan Press.[25]

In developing countries there has been an increase in dental decay experience. This has been particularly marked in the urban populations[27], which have greater access to more refined sugar products.

Periodontal disease

The distribution and trends in periodontal disease are more controversial due to problems in agreeing on common criteria for measuring disease. It is relatively difficult to identify the 10–15% of a population who are at risk of developing progressively destructive periodontal disease from the effects of poor oral hygiene.[28] Data at the WHO Global Bank demonstrate that the signs of poor oral hygiene – bleeding gums and calculus – are decreasing in industrialised societies. With oral hygiene generally poorer in developing countries[29], where dental resources are much scarcer, there is an obvious need for a preventive strategy aimed at improving an individual's oral health by encouraging more systematic mouth-cleaning habits. *Figure 1.7* summarises the current oral health trends and shows ratios of dental workers to population.

Tooth loss

The avoidance of tooth loss is the primary goal of dental health, and there have been major changes in many industrialised countries over recent decades.

Holistic Oral Care

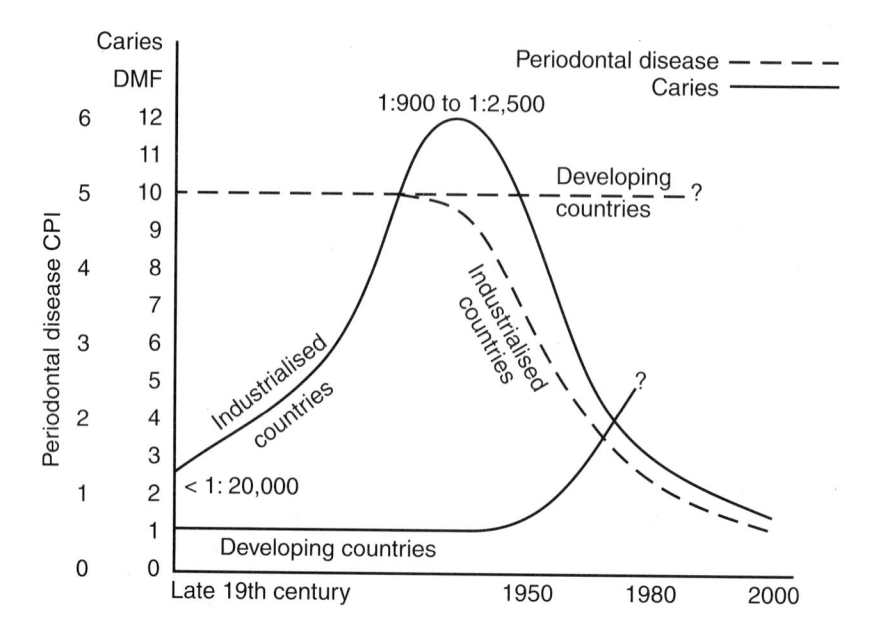

Figure 1.7 Oral health trends on a global basis using data at 12 years of age. By permission of Professor C.E. Renson.[28]

In the UK, the proportion of adults with some natural teeth rose from 70% in 1978 to 79% in 1988 and is expected to reach 90% by 2008. It is also expected that more than 90% of the working age population will be dentate with more than 21 teeth. There have been the most dramatic improvements in the dental health of young adults.[30] As a result of demographic changes and an increased life span, there will be increasing numbers of older people who are dentate.

For example, in the 55–64-year-old age group there has been a decrease in the number with no natural teeth from 56% in 1978 to 37% in 1988. It is reasonable to expect that these people will live longer and retain their teeth. The stereotypical view of the older person with full dentures will change radically over the next few decades and will force a considerable change in approaches to nursing care of the mouth. This will be discussed in greater depth in Chapter 4.

1.8 General Disability and Oral Handicap

In addition to the way in which a person's values, beliefs and environment can effect their oral health, the presence of any general disability may produce or worsen an oral handicap.

Oral Health and Disease

The major OPCS survey of disability[31] which examined the prevalence of disability in Britain looked at disability in terms of the functional effects upon daily living. The functions identified included:

- Locomotion.
- Dexterity.
- Hearing.
- Continence.
- Behaviour.
- Reaching and stretching.
- Seeing.
- Personal care.
- Communication.
- Intellectual functioning.

For most of these functions, disability will restrict or prevent a person carrying out those aspects of normal care necessary to maintain oral health. The extent to which disability may contribute to oral handicap is considerable with over six million adults in Britain above the threshold level of disability. Members of the health care team and carers need to be aware of the implications of disability in contributing to oral handicap. Section 3, especially Chapters 10, 11 and 12, will deal with disability from a functional viewpoint.

1.9 Phases in Prevention of Oral Disease and Oral Ill Health

Using the model of primary, secondary and tertiary prevention[32], there are a number of processes in which a partnership is essential between the dental team and other health workers.

Primary prevention
This is prevention before the appearance of any symptoms or disease, and also includes promoting positive health. In oral health, it involves:

- Establishing a well-balanced diet which is low in the sugars that produce dental caries.
- A reduction from the average 40kg of sugar consumption to 10–15kg per year.[33]
- Effective oral hygiene.
- Regular dental attendance.
- Encouraging positive values about good oral health.

The role of the primary health care professional is very evident when incorporating oral health into an holistic approach to good health.

Holistic Oral Care

Secondary prevention
At this stage there is already some disease present that will require arresting. But although there has been a failure of the primary preventive process, it is important to establish preventive regimes to limit the spread of further disease and return the person to good health. It is at this stage when they have experienced symptoms that many people seek out dental professionals.

Prevention at this stage can be particularly effective as the presence of existing disease can be a strong motivator to prevent further disease. Many people would not regard themselves as susceptible to disease, even though there may be predisposing factors in their lifestyle or environment. Other members of the health care team can identify early signs of disease and participate in maintenance programmes which help to minimise the spread of disease.

Tertiary prevention
At this stage, there is an established oral handicap which cannot be completely eradicated, and prevention is concerned with maintenance and maximising the remaining potential. Since other disabling conditions can compound oral handicap, there is an obvious need for a team approach to minimise unnecessary barriers.

1.10 Summary

Oral and dental disease consists of a number of conditions. The most important can be categorised as follows:

- Dental caries (dental decay) (*Colour Plates* **7, 8, 9, 10, 11**)
- Periodontal disease (gum disease) (*Colour Plates* **3, 4**)
- Oral infections (*Colour Plates* **21, 22 , 23, 24, 25**)
- Oral cancers (*Colour Plates* **28, 29, 30**)

Although dental caries and periodontal disease are caused by oral bacteria in dental plaque, there are many factors which will dictate whether, and how much, the individual is predisposed to these conditions.

These factors may be social, cultural or economic, and may determine sugar consumption, oral hygiene and access to dental services. Changes in these factors on a global, national or local level will alter the disease experience. Factors associated with oral cancers include occupation, use of tobacco in all forms, alcohol consumption and local factors.

The most effective form of dealing with oral and dental disease is a preventive strategy that involves the whole health care team.

1.11 References

1. Health Education Authority. (1989). *The most common disease in the world?*, DH19.
2. Health Education Authority. (1989). *The Scientific Basis of Dental Health Education*, 3rd ed., p. 4.
3. Smith, D.G. (1990). Primary prevention of periodontal disease. *Dent. Update*, Aug. **17** (6), 226–233.
4. Hindle, I. and Nally, F. (1991). Oral Cancer: a comparative study between 1962–7 and 1980–84 in England and Wales, *Br. Dental J.*, **170**(1), 15–24.
5. OPCS. (1978). *Occupational mortality*. The Registrar General's dicennial supplement for England and Wales, 1970–72. Series DS No. 1. London Office of Population Censuses and Surveys, HMSO.
6. Spitzer, W.O. *et al*. (1975). The occupation of fishing as a risk factor in cancer of the lip. *New Engl. J. Med.*, **293**, 419–424.
7. Binnie, W.H. and Rankin, K.V. (1988). Epidemiology of oral cancer. In: Wright, B.A., Wright, J.A. and Binnie, W.H. (eds), *Oral Cancer: Clinical and Pathological Considerations*. Florida, CRC Press pp. 2–11.
8. Preston-Martin, S, Henderson, B.E. and Pike, M. (1982). Descriptive epidemiol of cancers of the upper respiratory tract in Los Angeles. *Cancer*, **49**, 2201–2207.
9. Silverman, S. (1985). In: Silverman, S. (ed), *Oral Cancer*, New York American Cancer Society, pp. 2–6.
10. Wynder, E.L., Bross, I.J. and Feldman, R.M. (1957). A study of the etiological factors in cancer of the mouth. *Cancer*, **10**, 1300–1323.
11. Wynder, E.L., Mushinski, M.H. and Spirak, J.C. (1977). Tobacco and alcohol consumption in relation to the development of multiple primary cancers. *Cancer*, **40**, 1872–1878.
12. Smith, C.J. (1989). Oral cancer and precancer: Background, epidemiology and aetiology. *Br. Dent. Journal*. **167**, 377–383.
13. Pindborg, J.J. *et al*. (1971). Reverse smoking in Andhra Pradesh, India. A study of palatal lesions among 10,169 villagers. *Br. J. Cancer*, **25**, 10–20.
14. Hirayama, T. (1966). An epidemiological study of oral and oro-pharyngeal cancer in Central and South-East Asia. *Bull. WHO*, **38**, 41–69.
15. Wahi, P.N. (1968). The epidemiology of oral and oro-pharyngeal cancer: A study in Mainpuri District, Uttar Pradesh, India. *Bull. WHO*, **38**, 495–521.
16. Sundstrom, B., Mornstad, H. and Axell, T. (1982). Oral carcinomas associated with snuff dipping: some clinical and and histological characteristics of 23 tumours in Swedish males. *J. Oral Pathol.*, **11**, 245–251.
17. Herity, B., Moriarty, M., Bourke, G.J. and Daly, L. (1981). A case-control study of head and neck cancer in the Republic of Ireland. *Br. J. Canc.*, **43**, 177–182.
18. Lemon, F.R., Walden, R.T. and Woods, R.W. (1964). Cancer of the lung and mouth in Seventh-Day Adventists. Preliminary report on a population study. *Cancer*, **17**, 486–497.
19. Greenberg, R. S., Preston Martin, S., Bernstein, L., Schoenberg, J.B., Stemhagen, A. and Fraumeni, J. F. (1988). Smoking and drinking in relation to oral and pharyngeal cancer. *Cancer Res.*, **48**, 3282–3287.
20. Lowry, R. J. (1990). Prevention of oral carcinoma. *Dent. Update*, March, **17** (2), 58–61.
21. Cawson, R.A. and Binnie, W.H. (1980). *Candida*, leukoplakia and carcinoma: a possible relationship. In: Mackenzie, I.C., Dabelsteen, E. and Squier, C.A. (eds), *Oral Premalignancy*, Iowa City, University of Iowa Press.
22. Health Education Authority. *Do you take sugar?* DH 31. London, HEA.
23. Rugg-Gunn, A. (1990). Diet and Dental Caries. *Dental Update*, **17**(5), 198–201.

24. Rugg-Gunn. A. (1990). Prevention of Dental Caries. *Dental Update,* **17**(1), 24–27.
25. Evans, D.J. and Dowell, T.B. (1990). The dental caries experience of 12-year-old children in Great Britain. *Community Dental Health,* **7**(3), 307–314.
26. Bedi, R. and Elton, R.A. (1991). Dental caries experience and oral cleanliness of Asian and white Caucasian children aged 5–6 years attending primary schools in Glasgow and Trafford, UK. *Community Dental Health,* **8**(1), 18–23.
27. Olsson, B., Segura-Bernal, F. and Tanda, A. (1989). Dental caries in urban and rural areas in Mozambique. *Community Dental Health,* **6**(2), 139–147.
28. Renson, C.E. (1989). Global changes in caries prevalence and dental manpower requirements. 3. The effects on manpower needs. *Dental Update,* Nov., **16**(9), 382–389.
29. Matthesen, M., Baelum, V., Aarlsev, I. and Fejerskov, O. (1990). Dental health of children and adults in Guinea-Bissau, West Africa, in 1968. *Community Dental Health,* **7**(2), 123–135.
30. Downer, M.C. (1991). The improving dental health of United Kingdom adults and prospects for the future. *Br. Dent. J.,* **170**(4), 153–154.
31. Martin, J., Meltzer, H. and Elliot, D. (1988). *The Prevalence of Disability Among Adults: Report 1,* London, HMSO.
32. Ewles, L. and Simnett, I. (1987). *Promoting Health, a Practical Guide to Health Education,* Bristol, John Wiley, p. 17.
33. Sheiham, A. (1991). Why free sugars consumption should be below 15kg per person per year in industrialised countries: the dental evidence. *Br. Dent. J.,* **171**(2), 63–65.
34. Renson, C.E. (1989). Global changes in caries prevalence and dental manpower requirements: 2. The reasons underlying the changes in prevalence. *Dental Update,* **16**(8), 345–351.

2 Basic Principles and Practice of Oral Care

2.1 Introduction
2.2 Tooth care
2.3 Dietary care by reduction of refined sugars
2.4 Prevention of dental caries
2.5 Plaque control and the prevention of dental caries
2.6 The use of fluoride products
2.7 Dietary control of acids
2.8 Gum care
2.9 Mouth care
2.10 Malignant disease
2.11 Care of appliances
2.12 Denture use and abuse
2.13 Summary
2.14 References

2.1 Introduction

The introduction and opening chapter have set the scene for the reasons why primary health care professionals should be involved in oral care. The aim of this chapter is to set out the basic core principles and practices for oral care. A thorough grasp of the knowledge and skills in this section will enable any of the modifications described in later sections to be applied to the individual, in particular those with a special need.

As a starting point for the techniques necessary to maintain good oral health, the subject used will be a self-caring adult. For the average adult, there are three basic requirements, or social goals. These are:

- A functional set of teeth.
- A pleasing appearance.
- Freedom from discomfort and pain.

To achieve and maintain these goals, the individual requires a core of knowledge and health skills, motivation, the correct equipment (Chapter 9), and the opportunity and environment to put them into practice.

Holistic Oral Care

The basic knowledge and skills for oral care encompass five areas:

- Tooth care.
- Gum care.
- Mouth tissue care.
- Care of dentures and appliances (prostheses).
- Professional dental services (Chapter 5).

2.2 Tooth care

As outlined earlier, a number of factors are required for dental caries to occur. These can be best summed up by the following equation:

$$\text{Plaque} + \text{Sugar} \longrightarrow \text{Acid} + \text{Tooth Surface} \longrightarrow \text{Dental Caries}$$

The prevention of dental decay requires steps to be taken at all stages of the equation, including effective plaque removal from tooth surfaces, and strengthening the tooth surface to resist the effects of acid. The basic methods of prevention are in the hands of the self-caring adult, although professional help is also available. However, the single most effective step in preventing dental decay is to reduce the quantity and frequency of refined sugars.

2.3 Dietary care by reduction of refined sugars

The COMA report on *'Dietary Sugars and Human Disease'*[1] has reviewed the evidence in depth. The BDA supports these recommendations to prevent decay[2] (*Table 2.1*).

But if the evidence is so clear and the process seemingly so straightforward, why does the level of dental decay still constitute a major health problem? Some insight can be obtained if one considers the many reasons why and how refined sugars are consumed – the average amount consumed annually in the UK is 40kg per person.[3]

There are many strong social and cultural reasons why sugar and sugar-containing products are consumed.[4] Sugar is used as part of the celebration of most festivals, anniversaries and celebrations. It is used to console, reward, bribe and demonstrate affection. It is also used extensively as a preservative and as a bulking agent by the food industry.

Finally, and most importantly, society is subjected to intense and expensive persuasive advertising. The sugar multinationals spend many times the entire Health Education Authority's budget for dental health promotion on the launch of one confectionery bar![5] Is it so surprising

Table 2.1 Conclusions and recommendations from the COMA report on dietary sugars and human diseases.[1]

- Sugars are the most important dietary factor in the cause of dental caries. Caries experience is positively related to the amount of non-milk extrinsic sugars in the diet and the frequency of consumption.
- Dental caries can occur at any age, but those at greatest risk are children, adolescents and the elderly. Caries risk can be reduced by non-dietary means, particularly the use of fluoride, but these methods offer incomplete protection and some are expensive.
- The COMA panel recommends that consumption of non-milk extrinsic sugars by the population should be decreased. These sugars should be replaced by fresh fruit, vegetables and starchy foods.
- Those providing food for families and communities should seek to reduce the frequency with which sugary snacks are consumed.
- For infants and young children, simple sugars should not be added to bottle-feeds, sugared drinks should not be given in feeders where they may be in contact with the teeth for prolonged periods, dummies or comforters should not be dipped in sugars or sugary drinks.
- Older children need to be aware of the importance of diet and nutrition in relation to dental as well as general health. The panel recommends that schools should promote healthy eating patterns both by nutritional education and by providing and encouraging nutritionally sound food choices.
- Elderly people with teeth should restrict the amount and frequency of consumption of non-milk extrinsic sugars because their teeth are more likely to decay due to exposure of tooth roots and reduced salivary flow.
- The panel recommends that the Government should seek means to reduce the use of sugared liquid medicines. Parents and practitioners should select sugar-free alternatives where available.
- Dental practitioners should give dietary advice, including reduction of non-milk extrinsic sugars, as an important part of their health education, particularly to those prone to dental caries. The panel recommends that teaching of nutrition during dental training should be increased and professional relations between dietitians and dental practitioners be encouraged.

Source: adapted from Sections 14.3.1–14.3.9 of *Report on Health and Social Subjects 37*. By permission of the Controller of Her Majesty's Stationary Office.

that, when introduced to a pleasant-tasting substance at a very early age, which becomes associated with every pleasant occasion, and being cajoled constantly to consume it, many people find it idealistic to suggest that sugar consumption can be reduced and controlled? Yet many people are doing just that on a daily basis as part of calorie-controlled diets.

The frequent consumption of refined sugar-containing products is at the heart of the process which causes dental decay. The potential for producing dental caries seems to be greater with more refined rather than less refined sugars.[6] Thus, on a continuing spectrum, unrefined sugar cane and beet are less cariogenic (likely to contribute to dental caries or decay) than pulped sugar, which is less cariogenic than refined sugar – the most dangerous form of sugar for teeth.

The COMA report[1] does not define sugars in terms of their level of refinement, but in relation to their origin, as either intrinsic or extrinsic (*Table 2.2*). This information is of vital importance for the practical prevention of dental decay by dietary means. The substitution of dietary alternatives for refined or non-milk extrinsic sugar products reduces the risk of dental decay. It is obvious that occasional 'treats' pose little threat to our teeth, although the consumption of these 'treats' immediately after a meal is less harmful to teeth as it reduces the number of exposures to sugar.

Table 2.2 The COMA definition of sugar[1]

Intrinsic sugars

Sugars that form an integral part of certain unprocessed foodstuffs, the most important being whole fruits and vegetables. The sugars are enclosed within the plant cell and are mainly fructose, glucose and sucrose.

Extrinsic sugars

Sugars that are not located within the cellular structure of food. These fall into two groups:
- Milk sugars, which occur naturally in milk and milk products. These are almost entirely lactose, and are a negligible cause of dental decay, except under certain circumstances.
- Non-milk extrinsic sugars, which include fruit juices, honey and 'added sugars' (recipe and table sugars).

Careful examination of most refined foods reveals that sucrose has been added to many products, even the most unlikely, such as savoury sauces. Although these contribute to overall sugar consumption and contribute little more to the daily intake than 'empty calories' bereft of nutritional value, they do not pose the same risk to teeth as many snack

Basic Principles and Practice

products. By their very nature, snack foods are designed and marketed to be consumed between meals in convenient small portions, so increasing the number of 'acid attacks' on the teeth.

2.4 Prevention of dental caries

For the primary health care worker concerned with preventing dental decay, the first step is to gain a perspective of how much and how often sugar-containing products are consumed. A diet sheet which lists everything eaten over several days is a useful starting point (*Figures 2.1, 2.2*). The next step is to advise a gradual substitution to less damaging alternatives, and to suggest that sugar-containing products are less harmful if eaten at mealtimes. As a guide, *Table 2.3* lists less damaging alternatives to some common snacks.

Figure 2.1. Diet diary.

Choose a three-day period, either a Thursday, Friday and Saturday, or Sunday, Monday and Tuesday. Record everything eaten and drunk under the following headings.

The quantities should be as accurate as possible. It is very useful to record where the food was eaten or drunk, e.g. in the house, at school, at work, outside, and whether it was eaten alone, with friends, socially, etc.

Time	Food / Drink	Quantity	Eaten where	Doing
Day 1				
Day 2				
Day 3				

Figure 2.2. Diet sheet.

Write down in detail all the food and drink taken each day for *three days* (not consecutive), including everything consumed between meals. This will help to estimate the properties of the present diet.

Give the days of the week you choose and please include a Saturday or a Sunday. It is important that the times of meals and snacks are noted and whether any are eaten away from home, e.g. at school.

Suggested ways of measuring some of the foods

Food	Measure
Milk, orange juice, other drinks	in tablespoons, cups or tumblers
Breakfast cereals	in tablespoons
Bread	slices, large or small loaf, brown or white
Potatoes	in tablespoons or compare with an egg
Sugar	in teaspoons, dessert or tablespoons
Milk puddings, custard	in tablespoons
Biscuits	number and type
Jam, etc.	in teaspoons
Sweets, choc, ice cream	cost, size or number
Cod liver oil, vitamin supplements and over-the-counter medicines	in teaspoons

Day/time	Type of nourishment taken	Amount

Basic Principles and Practice

It is worth noting that the general principles of healthy eating, namely to reduce saturated fats, salt and sugar and increase dietary fibre, should be applied to any form of dietary advice. Viewing health holistically, it is not acceptable to replace a high-sugar product with a highly saturated-fat product.

Table 2.3 Alternative snack foods and drinks.

Snacks without added extrinsic sugars

- Fresh fruit
- Toast
- Crispy vegetables
- Crispbreads
- Natural yoghurt with fresh fruit
- Chapatis
- Unsweetened oatmeal biscuits
- Whole wheat bread
- Cottage cheese
- Pitta bread
- Low fat crisps
- Mashed banana
- Sugar-free peanut butter

Drinks without added extrinsic sugars

- Tea—without sugar
- Coffee—without sugar
- Herb tea—without sugar
- Plain lassi
- Semi-skimmed milk*
- Skimmed milk*
- Water, still or carbonated
- Diet carbonated drinks*
- Squashes with artificial sweetener*

* *Not recommended for children under two years old.*

2.5 Plaque control and the prevention of dental caries

Returning to the equation of the dental decay process, a prerequisite is bacterial plaque which with sugars produces the acid products that encourage demineralisation of the hard enamel surfaces of the teeth.

Examination of many people's mouths shows that dental decay has occurred in two main sites: the chewing surfaces of molar teeth (occlusal surfaces) and the surfaces between teeth known as the interproximal areas (*Figure 1.3*) (*Colour Plates* **8, 9**). These are the areas from which it is most difficult to remove plaque efficiently. It is difficult, if not impossible, to manipulate a toothbrush into the tiny crevices of the chewing surface. In addition, the process of demineralisation takes place within two minutes of consuming a suitable sugar. This considerably decreases the chance of plaque being removed before damage can occur.

It is important to practise good plaque control by brushing the teeth to remove all plaque and debris from the smooth surfaces and gum margins in order to prevent decay of these surfaces. However, there are other aids to plaque control besides a toothbrush. These consist of dental floss (*Figure 2.3*), a fine nylon cord or tape, and woodsticks. Both are used to clean in-between teeth. As a general principle, people should be taught individually by a dentist or dental hygienist how to use floss or woodsticks effectively.

Several mouthwashes appeared on the market recently claiming to improve plaque control by 'loosening' the plaque before brushing. There is still a lack of independent clinical trials to substantiate these claims.[7] The only chemical method of controlling plaque is by the use of gels, mouthwashes and sprays containing chlorhexidine, which is used in the control of gum disease and is considered later in this chapter and in Chapter 9.

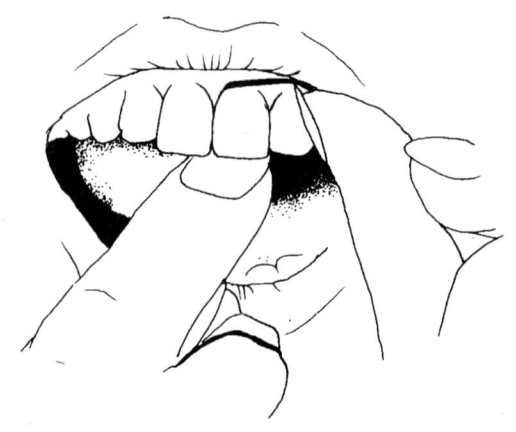

Figure 2.3 Flossing between incisor teeth

2.6 The use of fluoride products

Measures that strengthen the tooth's enamel surface can help create a surface which is more resistant to attack by acids. For the self-caring adult, this involves the application of fluoride-containing products directly to the surfaces of the teeth.

The simplest, cheapest and commonest method is by brushing with fluoride-containing toothpastes. The widespread use of such toothpastes has, over the last decade, been one of the major factors in the large reduction of dental decay in children.[8]

Fluoride supplements in the form of daily or weekly rinses can be self-administered.[9] Fluoride as a gel is usually applied by a member of the dental team, although a recently marketed product is available for individual use by toothbrushing. Fluoride supplements in the form of daily tablets and drops can produce significant reductions in dental decay in both the primary and secondary dentition (*Table 2.4*). The benefits are greatest when the supplements are used regularly from six months to 16 years, although smaller reductions in decay can be seen with a late start and irregular usage (Chapter 3).

Table 2.4 Dosage schedule for fluoride supplements (mgF/day).[9]

Age	Concentration of fluoride in drinking water		
	0.20	0.3–0.7	> 0.7
6 months–2 years	0.25	0	0
2–4 years	0.50	0.25	0
4–16 years	1.00	0.5	0

The most effective method of fluoride supplementation is by adjustment of the levels of fluoride in drinking water to one part per million. This is currently available to only 9% of the population, who demonstrate clear reductions in the level of dental caries of up to 55%. The greatest benefits are seen in children and in social classes IV and V, these groups being the least likely to attend the dentist for routine care.[8]

Progress in the fluoridation of public water supplies has been hindered by a variety of factors. The process of implementing the fluoridation of water supplies under the Water Fluoridation Act (1985) allows for extremely wide consultation with the population at all levels.[10] Despite the demonstrable benefits to the sectors of the community most at risk, a small vociferous lobby is able to delay implementation.

There is only the ethical issue of fluoridation which cannot be refuted by scientific enquiry. The core of the ethical argument for fluoridation is that it is unethical to deny other people its benefits, even if those benefits are not gained by all individuals, such as the self-caring adult not at risk from dental caries.

The only demonstrable side-effect of fluoride on teeth is enamel fluorosis which presents as mild opacities of the enamel surface. The benefits of fluoride to improved dental health undoubtedly outweigh the negligible effects of fluorosis. The Working Party which reviewed the epidemiological evidence on water fluoridation[11] concluded that there is no evidence to link fluoride and fluoridation with cancers and confirmed the safety of water fluoridation and continued monitoring of the evidence.

2.7 Dietary control of acids

Frequent consumption of food with a high acid content (*Table 2.5*) can lead to a more generalised loss of tooth enamel, sometimes affecting all the tooth surfaces. Some common drinks have a pH level of 2 or 3. The effect is to weaken the tooth surface. Certain foods or 'food addictions' (e.g. sucking lemons) often found in a healthy diet may confine this effect to a localised area. When combined with good oral hygiene, the surfaces of the teeth become highly polished and enamel is lost. The process of enamel loss is called erosion.

Table 2.5 Foods with a high acid content

- Lemons
- Vinegar
- Pickles
- Fruit juices
- Concentrated lemon juice

A careful analysis of the diet will usually identify the cause as due to frequent intake of fresh fruit or fruit juices. Changes in the diet, advice on correct tooth brushing techniques and topically applied fluoride are the most effective methods of preventing further damage. Acidic drinks consumed through a straw will reduce enamel exposure.

However, there are other rarer causes which are less easily controlled. Workers exposed to acid aerosols used regularly in some industrial processes may suffer enamel erosion. This occurs on the surfaces of the upper and lower anterior teeth, exposed during speech or when the lips are at rest. Individuals who suffer from frequent acid regurgitation, such as gastric illness, anorexia or bulimia, have an increased risk of developing erosion on the palatal surfaces of the teeth (*Colour Plate* **13**).

In both cases, fluoride is effective as a preventive measure. Soft, plastic, professionally constructed splints which fit over the surfaces of the teeth will help to protect the tooth enamel from exposure to atmospheric and gastric acids.

Basic Principles and Practice

2.8 Gum care

The major cause of tooth loss for adults is gum disease or chronic periodontal disease. The most effective method of prevention is the daily thorough removal of dental plaque from the gum margins.[9] The process of tooth loss can be summarised as follows:

Plaque —> Inflammation—> Gum Disease —> Tooth Loss

A self-caring adult can most effectively remove plaque using a systematic approach with a toothbrush and toothpaste. There are many different toothbrushing techniques, but there is no evidence to show that the simplest short scrubbing or rotary movements are any less effective. However, the 'sawing technique' when the necks of the teeth are brushed horizontally and vigorously can be harmful. This technique can create grooves in the necks of the teeth which may need to be filled (*Colour plate* **14**).

Similarly, there are many types of toothbrush available (*Figure 2.4*). The general guidelines are to select a small-headed brush with dense nylon filaments of a medium texture and to replace the brush when the

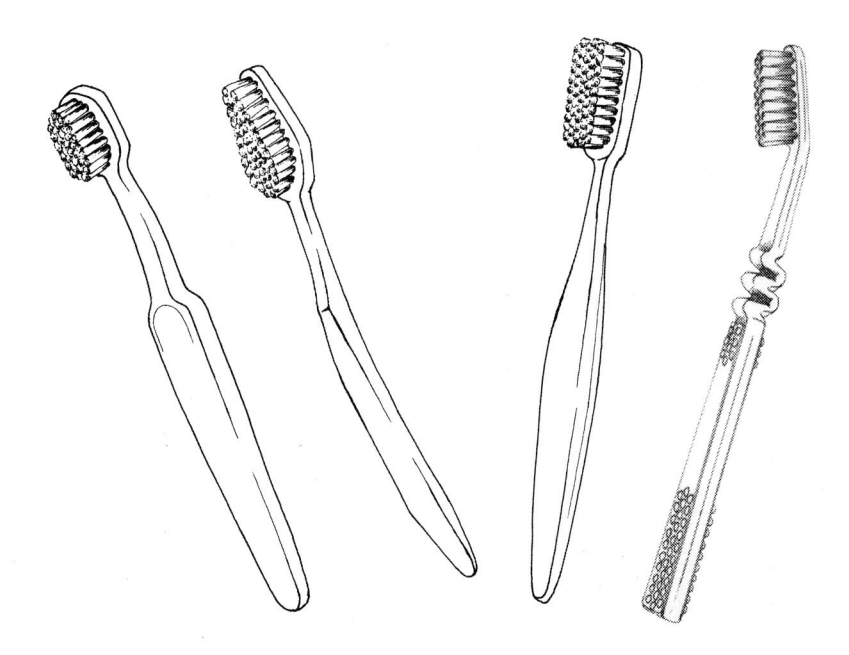

Figure 2.4. Toothbrushes.

filaments become 'splayed'. A variety of different heads may be advised for awkward areas. The shape of the handle is immaterial providing all surfaces of the teeth (cheek and palate and tongue side) can be reached. In order to achieve this, the compromise of a fairly straight handle is the most effective.

Once the filaments start to bend, a toothbrush is no longer effective in removing plaque and should be replaced. A toothbrush's average life is approximately three months in regular use. Travel toothbrushes which fold neatly away are useful when on the move. A dental hygienist is the best person to give advice on the most suitable toothbrush and the correct technique for each individual.

There are few guidelines for the selection of toothpaste. Provided the product contains fluoride the choice rests on individual taste, price and brand loyalty, although in rare cases allergy to toothpastes has been noted. Some toothpastes that claim to remove smoker's stains contain an abrasive which can literally 'polish' away the surfaces of the teeth. Other products that claim to whiten teeth do no more than dye the gums.

The British Dental Association has recently implemented a scheme whereby brands will be accredited with the Association's logo. Clinical claims made by the manufacturers have to be demonstrated in trials; these claims are examined by a panel of experts before being accepted as valid. Advertising is restricted to the accredited claims. This will help the public to make a more informed choice when buying oral care products.

Unfortunately, many people have an inefficient brushing technique. Thus where plaque has been allowed to accumulate, gum margins may become inflamed. These areas are more likely to bleed when brushed as any inflamed tissue is more friable. This is a very common finding.[12] Indeed, it is so common that most people do not even recognise it as a sign of disease and yet, at this stage, gums which bleed on brushing provide an early warning sign.

Healthy gums will not bleed following normal brushing and as such act as a useful indicator of the effectiveness of an individual's brushing technique. Even inflamed gums will respond to thorough brushing and return to a healthy condition following regular attention for a few days. *Colour Plate* **3** shows the appearance of gingivitis – the chronic inflammation of the gum margin or gingival tissue. Dental plaque in its early stages is invisible to the naked eye. The use of vegetable dyes in disclosing tablets or solutions highlights the areas where plaque has accumulated and can be a useful aid to oral care.

As well as regular brushing, the use of dental floss and woodsticks may be advised by an individual's dentist. This will improve the care of gums between teeth and around crowns and bridgework. Individual advice should be given on the use of floss and woodsticks.

The self-caring adult may occasionally need the temporary help with plaque control provided by chlorhexidine-containing mouth-care products. This usually forms part of an active course of dental treatment and long-term use of these products is not recommended due to the side-effect of staining the teeth. However, teeth can be professionally polished to remove stains far more easily than gum disease can be cured.

2.9 Mouth care

The only other regular care required by a self-caring adult for tissues in the mouth, apart from the gums, is a gentle sweeping action to brush the inside of the cheeks, the surface of the tongue and the palate. This can also be carried out with a finger wrapped in gauze. Vigorous rinsing is effective to ensure no food particles are retained. Mouth care should be practised by individuals who are edentulous (with no natural teeth) as much as by individuals who are dentate (with some or all of their natural teeth).

Any tissues normally covered by dentures or other removable mouth appliances should be thoroughly rinsed with plain water and gently brushed, after the appliance has been removed, to ensure that no food particles have been retained and to remove plaque. The denture should also be brushed with a toothbrush or denture brush and rinsed in cold water before being replaced in the mouth.

Antiseptic mouthwashes and gargles only give a very short-term sensation of cleanliness. There is little evidence to show that they have any benefits.[13]

2.10 Malignant disease

It is worth briefly considering other behaviours known to affect oral health. Some habits of the self-caring individual are known causative factors in oral malignant disease; the risks of tobacco in all its forms[14] are described in Chapter 1. Occupational groups with easy access to alcohol have a greater incidence of oral cancers, as shown in French workers employed in the wine industry. The combination of both tobacco and alcohol greatly increases the risk of oral cancers.[15]

Counselling to change high-risk health behaviour is outside the scope of this book, but good oral hygiene and regular oral screening as part of a routine check-up by a dentist for early diagnosis of premalignant and malignant conditions must be recommended.

2.11 Care of appliances

The types of appliance that the self-caring adult may wear in her or his mouth fall into two main categories: removable and fixed. All appliances collect plaque and food debris and, although the methods of cleaning may vary, the general principles for removing plaque apply to all forms of appliance.

Fixed appliances
These are semi-permanently or permanently attached to the teeth and should only be removed by a member of the dental profession. By definition, these must be cleaned in the mouth and greater care must be taken to ensure the effective control of plaque. Individual tuition in oral care is usually provided when the appliance is fitted. Fluoride mouthwashes and chemical plaque control may be advised as added preventive measures. Fixed appliances include:
- Bridges to replace missing teeth.
- Orthodontic appliances cemented to the teeth.
- Wiring following jaw fractures or maxillofacial surgery.

Bridges
For people with dental bridges or more complex types of appliances which are permanently or semi-permanently in the mouth, individual cleaning instruction is essential. The same principles apply as to the care of natural teeth, i.e. thorough cleaning with a toothbrush and the use of dental floss. Disclosing solutions are very useful to indicate the areas where plaque accumulates around fixed appliances. Professional advice on oral care is generally provided for the individual's specific needs. The dental hygienist has an important role in providing individual advice and tuition.

Orthodontic appliances
A fixed orthodontic appliance, commonly known as a 'brace', and which may carry complex wires and springs, is cemented to the surfaces of teeth. It requires very thorough cleaning with a soft toothbrush to ensure that all plaque and debris are removed. Professional oral hygiene advice is again recommended.

Fixation
Caring for a mouth which has been fixed with wiring following a fracture or surgery poses obvious problems for the efficient removal of dental plaque and debris. Even though the person may be nourished by a liquid

Basic Principles and Practice

or semi-liquid diet, he or she will still be at risk from dental decay. In addition, the difficulty of maintaining healthy gums will increase the level of oral discomfort.

The primary health worker may seek advice from the dental hygienist but the general principles remain the same. In addition to thorough careful brushing and dietary control of sugars, chlorhexidine-containing products may be used to control plaque, and chlorhexidine mouthwash can be given through a straw (Chapters 9 and 16).

Removable appliances
These can and should be removed for thorough cleaning. They include:

- Full dentures.
- Partial dentures.
- Orthodontic appliances ('braces').
- Removable bridges.
- Obturators (to restore a cleft palate).
- Other prostheses replacing hard and soft tissues.

Dentures
The commonest removable appliances worn in the UK are dentures.[16] These should be removed after eating and rinsed clean. They should be cleaned thoroughly each day with a soft brush and ordinary unperfumed household soap. This should be done over a basin of cold water to prevent breakage if the dentures are accidentally dropped.

Partial dentures and appliances with wires or clasps are more prone to collect food and need more attention. It is worthwhile stressing the importance of thorough cleaning of support teeth next to the partial dentures and teeth which support clasps or wires.

Hard deposits that form on removable appliances occur as a result of calcium deposits in plaque. Deposits mainly form on the cheek side of the upper denture and near the base of the tongue on the lower denture. These hard deposits, called tartar or calculus, should be removed professionally before the roughened denture surface causes irritation and inflammation. Staining may also occur due to tobacco or the effect of certain food and drink, e.g. tea and coffee. Poor denture hygiene is often associated with oral candidal infections.

Removable orthodontic appliances
These should be cleaned very carefully so as not to damage wires and springs. The orthodontist may have instructed that the appliance should be worn at night; plaque must be thoroughly removed from both teeth and appliance.

Holistic Oral Care

Obturators and facial prostheses
These appliances are individually constructed to close cleft palates or to replace missing hard and soft tissues following maxillofacial surgery. They require the same basic care as dentures but any specific professional advice should be followed.

2.12 Denture use and abuse

Care of dentures
Whether an appliance should be worn at night depends upon the type of appliance and the advice given when it is fitted. All appliances, when not worn, should be immersed in water to prevent the distortion that occurs when plastic appliances are allowed to dry out. Hot water should be avoided for the same reasons.

Generally, all dentures should be left out of the mouth at night. Prolonged and repeated night use, particularly if dentures are not plaque-free may lead to oral infections, such as oral candidiasis (thrush) (*Colour Plates* **22, 23**). These infections frequently go unnoticed until they becomes acute. If dentures are worn at night, then they must be scrupulously clean and the wearer must be made aware of the potential risks of this practice.

Self-applied commercial soft linings and denture fixatives should not be used as they may mask existing problems which should be dealt with professionally. These linings act as a medium for the rapid proliferation of micro-organisms, in particular fungae. Denture fixatives should only be used as a temporary measure or on the advice of a dentist.

A dry mouth (xerostomia) may be the cause of poor denture retention. If dentures are loose or ill-fitting, then a visit to the dentist is advisable. It is worth noting that the life expectancy of dentures is approximately five years, and yet many people believe that they last longer, some thinking for the rest of their lifetime (*Colour Plate* **32**).

Professionally fitted soft linings can dramatically improve comfort for some individuals who experience persistent discomfort in wearing dentures due to resorption of the bony ridges. Soft linings have a limited life; they gradually lose their elasticity and usually require replacement within about two years. Professional advice on care should be given at the time of fitting to ensure that maximum resilience is retained.

Denture hygiene
Denture cleaners may be effective in removing staining, but long-term submersion is not indicated as these products may have a bleaching action, which will discolour the denture and may damage any special linings. Special care is needed to clean soft linings in order to prevent

Basic Principles and Practice

them hardening prematurely. The resilience of the soft lining may be affected by denture cleaning materials and the heat of the water used.

Most proprietary denture cleaners, whether solutions, brush-on cleaners or pastes, have some disadvantages (*Table 2.6*). Rinsing or soaking dentures does not remove plaque efficiently; as with teeth, brushing is the most effective method of removing plaque. Regular brushing with unperfumed soap and water is now considered to be the best method of cleaning dentures, although proprietary cleaners may at times be recommended. The subjective impression of freshness which may be provided by some proprietary denture cleaners should not be discounted.

Soaking dentures in a chlorhexidine mouthwash is effective in reducing plaque, although dentures may become stained. Some effervescent cleaners can be mistaken for sweets, as in the case of the accidental death of an elderly person in hospital.[17]

Table 2.6 Denture cleaners.

Denture cleaner	Method	Effect
Alkaline peroxides	Soaking	Do not readily remove stain
Hypochlorite	Soaking	May cause bleaching
		May corrode metal dentures
		Removes plaque well
Chlorhexidine	Soaking	May stain dentures
		Very effective against plaque
Dilute acids	Brush on	Effective for stain removal and heavy deposits
		May corrode metal dentures
Denture pastes	Brushing	Abrasive to denture plastic

Ultrasonic cleaning baths can be obtained from most dental equipment suppliers, and are useful for removing hard deposits which otherwise could only be removed professionally. In hospitals and residential care, this equipment can provide a professional denture-cleaning service for patients and residents. It is advisable to name dentures beforehand to ensure that dentures are returned to their rightful owner.

Naming dentures

Labelling dentures with the owner's name is a very sensible but fairly recent practice. The name is only visible when the dentures are removed and the process is easily carried out during the laboratory construction of dentures. Older dentures are unlikely to be named in this way, but can be named after construction. Individuals who wish to have their dentures named should ask their dentist for this service. Temporary marking can be protected by nail varnish but it is not very durable.

A commercially produced kit, 'Identure', is sufficient for naming large numbers of dentures. It can generally be purchased from dental suppliers, and is particularly useful for hospitals, nursing and residential homes. It can also be used for naming plastic spectacles.

Anecdotal evidence about the communal cleaning of dentures is fortunately now rare. However, the authors have been called upon to identify unnamed dentures which have become confused during communal cleaning. Identifying the owner of dentures in such cases can be difficult or impossible, even for an experienced dentist.

2.13 Summary

For the self-caring adult, the basic principles and practice of oral care are elementary. The difficulties lie in that most people receive their knowledge from a wide variety of conflicting sources and follow habits and routines established over many years, which are difficult to modify and make more effective.

Many self-caring adults do not visit the dentist except when the need arises[18], and thus do not have the most up-to-date advice on oral care. It is therefore not surprising that misbeliefs about the inevitability of tooth loss and the life expectancy of dentures are still so prevalent.

When other health threats upset self-care routines, personal and oral care may suffer. As most people have never learnt oral care in a systematic manner based on scientific evidence, there is often potential for improvement (*Figure 2.5*).

2.14 References

1. COMA. Department of Health. (1989). *Dietary Sugars and Human Disease*. Report of the Panel on Dietary Sugars of the Committee on Medical Aspects of Food Policy. Report No 37. London, HMSO.
2. Editorial. (1990). *Br. Dent. J.*, **168**(2), 45–47.
3. Health Education Authority. (1988) *Do you take sugar?* DH31. London, HEA.
4. Davis, P. (1987). *Introduction to the sociology of dentistry*. Otago Press, p. 58.
5. Sarll, D. (1990). The politics of sugar. *Community Dental Health*, **7**(4), 347–349.
6. Rugg-Gunn, A.J. (1990). Diet and dental caries. *Dental Update*, June, **17**(5), 198–201.
7. Addy, M. (1989). Pre-brushing mouthrinse, Plax. (Letter). *Br. Dent. J.*, **167**(1), 10–11.
8. Rugg-Gunn, A.J. and Murray, J.J. (1990). Current issues in the use of fluorides in dentistry. *Dental Update*, **17**(4), 154–158.
9. Levine, R.S. (1989). *The Scientific Basis of Dental Health Education*. 3rd Ed. London, Health Education Authority.
10. British Fluoridation Society. (1985). *Making Decisions on Water Fluoridation*. London, BFS, p. 4.

Basic Principles and Practice

11. Knox, E.G. (Chairman). (1985). *Fluoridation of Water and Cancer: A Review of the Epidemiological Evidence. Report of the Working Party.* London, HMSO.
12. Smith, D.G. Primary prevention of periodontal disease. 1990 *Dental Update*, July/Aug., 226–232.
13. Hogg, S.D. (1990). Chemical control of plaque. *Dental Update*, Oct., 330–334.
14. Lowry, R.J. (1990). Prevention of oral carcinoma. *Dental Update*, Mar., 58–61.
15. Greenberg, R.S., Preston Martin, S., Bernstein, L., Schoenberg, J.B., Stemhagen, A. and Fraumeni, J.F. (1988). Smoking and drinking in relation to oral and pharyngeal cancer. *Cancer Research*, **48**, 3282–3287.
16. Todd, J.E. and Lader, D. (1991). *Adult Dental Health 1988.* London, OPCS, Social Survey Division, HMSO.
17. Mackenzie, I.J. (1982). A denture cleansing tablet swallowed. *Br. Dent. J.*, **153**, 6–7.
18. Todd, J.E. and Lader, D. (1991). *Adult Dental Health 1988.* U.K. p.217. HMSO.

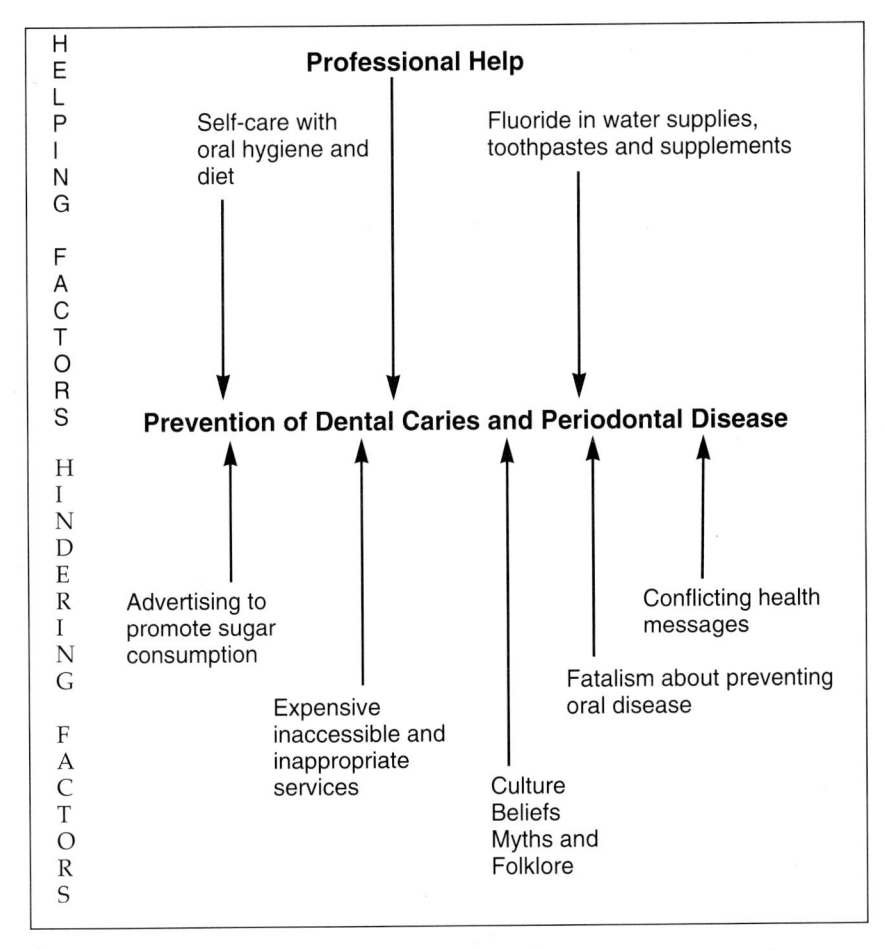

Figure 2.5. Helping and hindering factors in oral care

3 Child Dental Health

3.1 Children as a special group
3.2 The need to establish primary prevention in childhood
3.3 The primary and secondary dentition
3.4 The process for an oral preventive strategy
3.5 Phase 1: Assessment
3.6 Phase 2: Planning an holistic approach to prevention
3.7 Phase 3: Action. Implementing practical preventive regimes for children
3.8 Oral Hygiene Measures
3.9 Phase 4: Evaluation
3.10 Summary
3.11 References

3.1 Children as a special group

Traditionally, children have been identified as a special group, which is more 'at risk' from dental and oral disease. This is due to society's perception of the dependent status of children, who, as a group, require special protection and provisions. In addition, the onset of dental disease during childhood in most industrialised societies results in a focus on children as a target group for primary prevention.

A number of socio-demographic changes underway will change these assumptions. The changing age structures in most industrialised countries will mean that the number and proportion of older people will increase as the number and proportion of children declines.[1] Indeed, it is the older population who will pose the greatest treatment challenges to both the dental profession and health care teams. However, this should not detract from the vital importance of preventing oral and dental disease during childhood.

The initial high prevalence of dental disease in children leads to a focusing of dental services and an allocation of resources on this group by many countries.[2] However, the reduction in the prevalence of dental caries seen in many industrialised societies will significantly reduce the overall treatment needs of children. But, due to the strong association of dental disease with aspects of deprivation and with socio-economic factors, the focus will pass to different subgroups of children in the community, to those identified as being more at risk than the whole group of children *per se*.

Child Dental Health

The social, cultural and environmental aspects of dental disease may place children more at risk as dental caries begins with the widespread use throughout childhood of sugar and sugar-containing products as a pacifier, bribe or reward. Snacking between meals, which increases the risk of caries, is also part of the youth culture.[3]

In developing countries, the caries rate is rising in those parts of the community with access to refined sugar products.[4] Although children are predominently affected, the whole community is at risk once the challenge to dental health of increased sugar has been introduced. All health care professionals need to recognise the limitations of labelling children as a group with greater inherent susceptibility to dental disease, in isolation of social factors.[5] These factors include exposure to fluoride in water and/or toothpastes, dietary patterns, use of dental services, and the degree to which families or communities value a preventive approach to oral health.

3.2 The need to establish primary prevention in childhood

The patterns of dental treatment needs and an individual's attitude to oral health are shaped by childhood experiences. The routines established during childhood, in the phase of primary socialisation[6] will form the basis of many of our adult behaviour patterns. The stress and anxiety that many adults suffer are the result of traumatic dental visits in childhood, often involving the extraction of primary teeth under a general anaesthetic.[7] Early experience of dental caries and any subsequent treatment will map out a person's treatment needs throughout adult life, as fillings wear out and require periodic replacement. As restorations are replaced, inevitably they become larger and need more complex replacements. A person's future needs can be largely predicted from the state of their oral health when 12–14 years old.[8]

3.3 The primary and secondary dentition

There are a number of anatomical differences between the primary and secondary dentition, but these do not intrinsically alter the susceptibility to dental caries. It is important for all health professionals to encourage a preventive approach, even during that part of a child's life when the primary dentition is present. Active prevention and treatment of any dental caries on primary teeth is necessary for the following reasons:

- To prevent pain.
- To reduce the need for extractions.
- To prevent orthodontic complications in the secondary dentition[9] (*Colour Plate* **15**).

Early experiences of dental-related pain and subsequent treatment which may involve extraction of teeth will strongly contribute to producing a dentally anxious patient.[10] Early loss of primary teeth may also encourage the following secondary teeth to erupt in unfavourable positions, which can result in poor aesthetics. Crowded and malpositioned teeth will additionally be more difficult to clean effectively (*Colour Plate* **15**).

Although the crowns of the primary teeth are all fully developed at birth, the secondary teeth start to calcify around this time (*Figures 3.1, 3.2*). Birth or perinatal trauma can even produce a distinctive 'line' visible, when the permanent incisor teeth erupt into the mouth at around 6–7 years.

Untreated dental decay in the primary teeth can damage the developing secondary teeth and result in malformations and damage to the permanent teeth developing underneath.

3.4 The process for an oral preventive strategy

Whichever method is used for planning and implementing a preventive strategy, it is important to use a logical, planned approach, similar to the cyclical nursing process:assessement, planning, implementation and evaluation.

3.5 Phase 1: Assessment

In most cases this will take place in an interview with the parent or parent substitute. The first steps in establishing sound preventive behaviour during childhood will depend very strongly on the attitudes and beliefs of the parent or guardian. Their past experiences can sometimes result in a conflict between a wish for their children to avoid their own experiences, and a fatalism that their children will inevitably suffer dental disease.[11]

There are many variables that affect health-related behaviour; these can be sociological or part of the individual's psychological make-up.[12] It

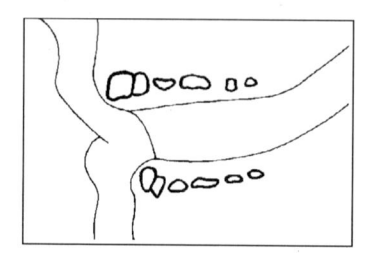

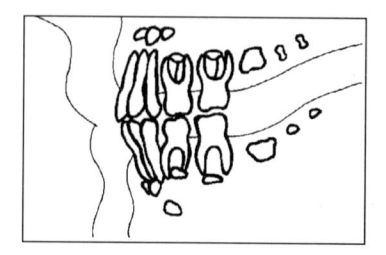

Figure 3.1 (left). Primary teeth developing in the jaws of an unborn child.

Figure 3.2 (right). Secondary teeth developing behind the primary teeth. There is no primary tooth preceding the first permanent molar.

is understandable that parents might wish to avoid their child suffering pain and discomfort. But this, coupled with a negative attitude to the value of prevention and regular dental attendance, can encourage an avoidance of dental visits, except for acute problems.

There is a tendency to predict individuals' views by assuming that they hold the views of their socio-economic group. For example, it is commonly believed that people from low socio-economic groups are fatalistic about their health and see little value in prevention.[13] However, other more detailed examinations of groups show that more complex reasoning is taking place, based on the values of the family network, individual trust in health services and professionals, and past treatment experience.[14] Indeed, because of the complexity of predicting behaviour, it is better for the health professional to approach the practical situation with as few preconceptions as possible. It is in contact with the dental services that other members of the health care team have a vital role in overcoming the anxiety barrier.

3.6 Phase 2: Planning an holistic approach to prevention

Much of our health service is organised like a departmental store, with separate sections for different organs, diseases and processes. This reflects the views of the health professions about the body being like a machine with different components, rather than the everyday view of 'health' involving both the body and the mind.

This separation into specialities extends into prevention and can become a barrier. Although it is reasonable to expect specialisation into different complex areas of medical interventions, the reason for the specialised division of labour becomes less clear in preventive strategies.

The actual core messages of, and approaches to, prevention of dental disease should be incorporated into the preventive aspects practised by all involved in health care. While the knowledge of, and techniques for, the diagnosis and treatment of dental and oral disease remain a specialised area in many countries, primary prevention will only be more successful when presented as part of a total 'package' by all members of the health team.

Detecting the 'at-risk' individual

As described in Chapter 1, there is a general downward trend in dental disease in children in industrialised societies. However, there are still groups and individuals substantially at risk within particular communities. It is in these groups that most dental disease is becoming concentrated. As well as a 'whole population' approach to prevention, additional support is necessary for those at higher risk.

The success of this approach lies in identifying higher-risk individuals through careful questioning and consultation. Those children more at risk may include groups who experience additional barriers. These will be considered in more depth in Section 3, but an overview reveals several broad groups as discussed below.

Medical conditions

The presence of other medical conditions may place a child more at risk from the effects of dental treatment. Long-term medication for children is often delivered in syrup form to make it more palatable. Although sugar-free alternatives to many paediatric syrups are available, these are not always prescribed (Chapter 8). Chronically 'sick' children may also be more at risk, as good dental health may be considered a low priority by parents, guardians or other health professionals.

Physical or mental disabilities

Unfortunately, there are still widespread perceptions that children with a learning disability are unable to receive routine dental care. Consequently, they may have delayed contact with the preventive aspects of the dental service. This is also true of children with a physical disability, for whom environmental barriers exist. Furthermore, the stress and pressures of caring for a disabled child may encourage over-protection, comforting with sweetened foods and sweets, and the avoidance of potentially stressful situations, such as dental attendance.

Social group

There are inherent problems in predicting behaviour according to how health professionals perceive a particular social group or class should behave. But there is no doubt that a greater understanding of an individual's social circumstances will help formulate a more suitable preventive approach. Using careful non-judgemental questioning, it is possible to ascertain the individual's current views and knowledge, which can act as a foundation on which to build. This will include an assessment of the value of oral health and the dental attendance pattern of the parent or guardian.

Geographical location

Although closely related to social class, the presence of other children, work commitments and poor public transport may create barriers which influence preventive regimes. The availability and types of local shopping can affect the provision of a healthy diet.

Presence of existing dental disease

Although a detailed diagnosis remains the domain of the dental professional, Section 2 of this guide will help to provide pointers that indicate a more detailed oral examination is required. Unfortunately, it may be only too obvious even to the untrained eye that there is existing dental caries (*Colour Plates* **7, 8, 9**).

Summary and interpretation of high-risk assessment

Figure 3.3 provides a summary of assessment and interpretation of five areas of data used in assessing the caries risk of individuals.[15]

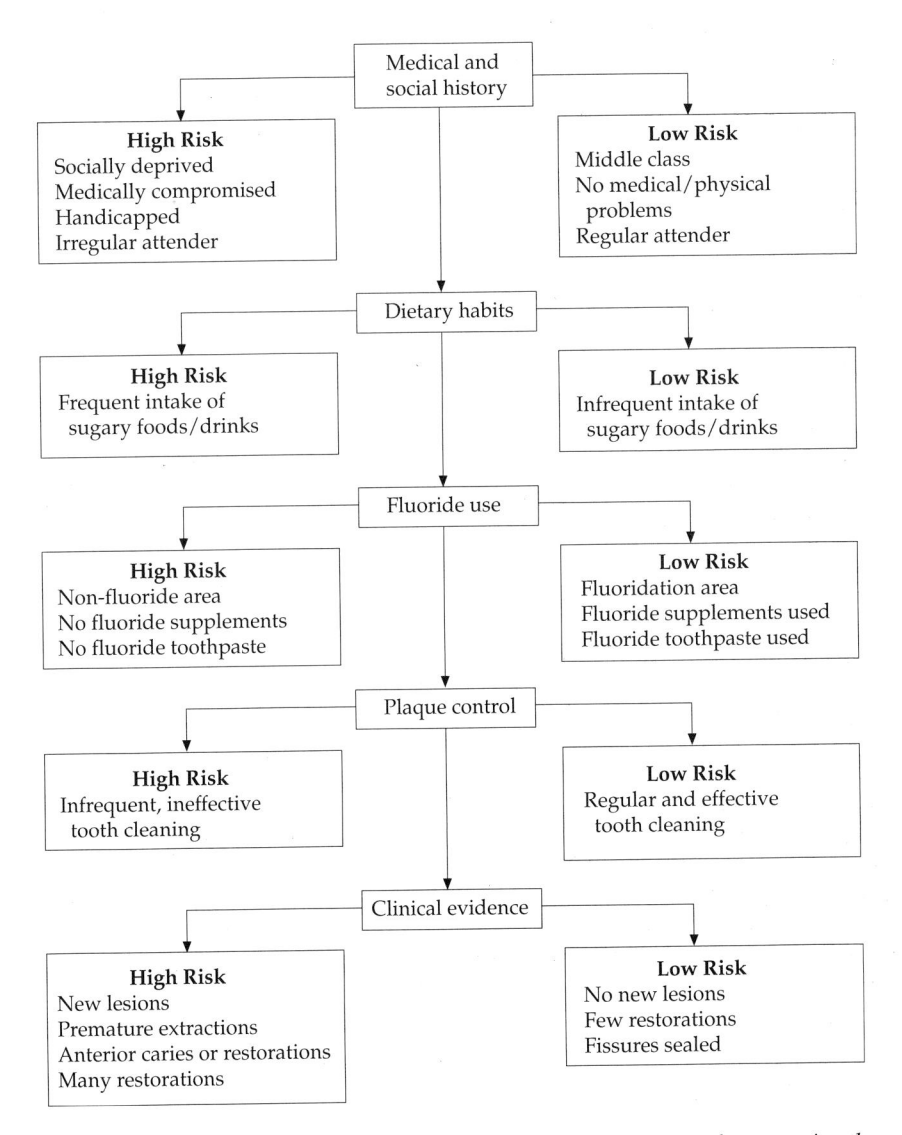

```
                    Medical and
                    social history

High Risk                              Low Risk
Socially deprived                      Middle class
Medically compromised                  No medical/physical
Handicapped                              problems
Irregular attender                     Regular attender

                    Dietary habits

High Risk                              Low Risk
Frequent intake of                     Infrequent intake of
  sugary foods/drinks                    sugary foods/drinks

                    Fluoride use

High Risk                              Low Risk
Non-fluoride area                      Fluoridation area
No fluoride supplements                Fluoride supplements used
No fluoride toothpaste                 Fluoride toothpaste used

                    Plaque control

High Risk                              Low Risk
Infrequent, ineffective                Regular and effective
  tooth cleaning                         tooth cleaning

                    Clinical evidence

High Risk                              Low Risk
New lesions                            No new lesions
Premature extractions                  Few restorations
Anterior caries or restorations        Fissures sealed
Many restorations
```

Figure 3.3 Flow diagram showing five types of data to be considered when assessing the caries risk of individual patients.[15] Reproduced by permission of Butterworth Heineman.

3.7 Phase 3: Action. Implementing practical preventive regimes for children

Having established the degree of risk, the key to success is to make a number of small changes over a period of time, rather than attempting drastic alterations in routines which will not be maintained.

Dietary changes

Particularly for children with active dental caries, it is important to identify the number of sugar intakes. These include not only those in confectionery and added sugar, but also 'hidden' in fruit squashes and carbonated drinks. Snack foods and drinks are high in sugar content.

Since it is the frequency or number of sugar intakes which is crucial in the development of dental caries, a suitable strategy is the restriction of any sugar-containing products to mealtimes. A particularly high-risk time for children is at night when they may be given a sugary drink in a feeder or a sugar-dipped dummy.

Sugar is sometimes added to bottle-feeds in the belief that the child will benefit from the extra calories, and the lay belief still persists that sugar in water is a remedy for constipation. The distinctive pattern of decay on the front teeth caused by contact with sugar solutions, often referred to as 'bottle caries', can be seen in *Colour Plate* 7. Due to conflicting information received from media advertising and unclear labelling, parents frequently fail to appreciate the hidden sugar content of foods and drinks. There are also long-standing erroneous views that certain products are safer for children's teeth, for example that white chocolate is less cariogenic than ordinary chocolate.

The other key strategy is the use of sugar substitutes in the diet. This refers not just to the use of artificial sweeteners, but also to the use of rewards, such as toys, comics or books, instead of sweets or other sweet-tasting foods. Artificial sweeteners are not recommended for children under two years old as they may cause gastric problems.

More detailed lists of sugar substitutes can be found in Appendix 1. Sugar in drinks and confectionery form a significant part of the dietary intake for all groups[16], none more so than young adults for whom consumption of such products is part of youth culture (*Colour Plates* 8, 9). Decisions in youth, including patterns of sugar consumption, are very strongly affected by peer group pressure, which can override an individual's intentions not to consume sugar on dental health grounds.[17] This desire to conform is used extensively in the advertising of sugar-containing drinks and confectionery, which often portray models using these products.

Child Dental Health

3.8 Oral hygiene measures

Toothbrushing

There are two main reasons for toothbrushing:

- To remove plaque to prevent dental caries and periodontal disease.
- To apply a daily dose of fluoride topically to the teeth.

This is of course the rationale for toothbrushing from a medical perspective, while most individuals have the social goals of wanting clean teeth and fresh breath, as part of the grooming process.[18]

The twice-daily brushing of teeth varies considerably throughout countries, communities and gender, as reflected in *Table 3.1*.[19] The variation can be partly explained by family socialisation patterns which may be very resistant to change. Other factors, such as family size and social class, can influence the

Table 3.1 The twice daily brushing of teeth by gender, social class, and community in ten study areas.

Study area		% of students brushing their teeth twice or more						
		Male Social Position			Female Social Position			
		Low	High	Total	Low	High	Total	Total
Baltimore	Metro	46	48	47	60	65	63	55
	Nonmetro	37	46	44	60	77	72	57
Ontario	Metro	51	70	60	76	86	80	70
	Nonmetro	44	67	55	75	87	79	67
Sydney	Metro	62	70	68	76	84	82	74
	Nonmetro	47	73	68	78	88	84	77
Hannover	Metro	58	68	64	75	84	79	71
	Nonmetro	56	71	62	85	92	87	75
Yamanashi	Metro	14	28	24	31	43	39	31
	Nonmetro	7	13	11	21	21	21	16
Canterbury	Metro	51	60	58	61	76	73	66
	Nonmetro	42	56	52	65	74	71	61
Dublin	Metro	33	42	35	63	75	68	51
	Nonmetro	37	63	45	63	75	70	58
Trondelag	Metro	60	80	68	85	95	89	78
	Nonmetro	58	69	62	86	88	87	74
Leipzig	Metro	69	80	73	91	91	91	82
	Nonmettro	68	76	70	83	92	87	79
Lodz	Metro	34	39	38	58	74	70	53
	Nonmetro	21	30	25	32	48	42	34

Source: World Health Organisation. Oral Health Care Systems, an international collaborative study coord. by WHO (1985), by permission of Quintessence Publishing Co Ltd.

frequency of toothbrushing among children and particularly adolescents.[20] As part of the assessment phase the 'when and where' aspects of oral hygiene behaviour need to be established, who has responsibility for supervising toothbrushing in the home, and how it fits into the domestic routine.

Techniques for effective toothbrushing are the same for a child as for an adult (Chapter 2). The main difference is that children up to the age of seven will require help, particularly in the posterior regions of the mouth, and the surfaces next to the tongue and palate.

As part of the socialisation process, it is important that young individuals have the opportunities to acquire and practise skills for themselves. Toothbrushing therefore becomes part teaching and part supervisory, as the child becomes more proficient (*Figures 3.4–3.6*).

For toothbrushing to be effective in preventing dental disease, a small number of thorough brushings are better than frequent, scant brushing. There is little to be gained from brushing after every meal, and for most children this would not be practical in many school environments.

Other hygiene techniques

The use of dental floss can aid in removing plaque from between teeth. It does require a high level of manual dexterity and considerable practice before it can be used comfortably. Dentists who are used to working intra-orally and with mirrors may underestimate the difficulty. Children do not really develop the required level of dexterity to use floss safely until about 12 years of age. The use of floss should be taught on an individual basis by a member of the dental team and practised under supervision, as misuse can damage gum tissue.

The use of fluorides

The simplest, most effective way of administering fluoride is via the drinking water supply. This method has been shown to be safe and effective in literally hundreds of studies carried out since the first city, Grand Rapids, USA, received fluoridated water in 1945.[21]

The next most important source of fluoride is via toothpaste. It is more difficult to control the amount of fluoride ingested with young children; only a 'pea-sized' amount should be used and the child should be encouraged to rinse and spit out. This will avoid the risk of 'mottling' or fluorosis of the enamel in the permanent teeth.[22]

The same level of protection as that given by water fluoridation can be conferred by systemic fluoride supplements. These are as drops for the youngest age group and tablets (and mouth rinses) for older children. However, it is difficult to ensure that children keep taking a daily dose for a prolonged period, until the permanent teeth are fully formed at approximately seven years of age. If the regime is continued until all the teeth have erupted into the mouth in early adolescence, then extra protection will be given as the enamel continues to mature and is able to take up the extra fluoride.

Child Dental Health

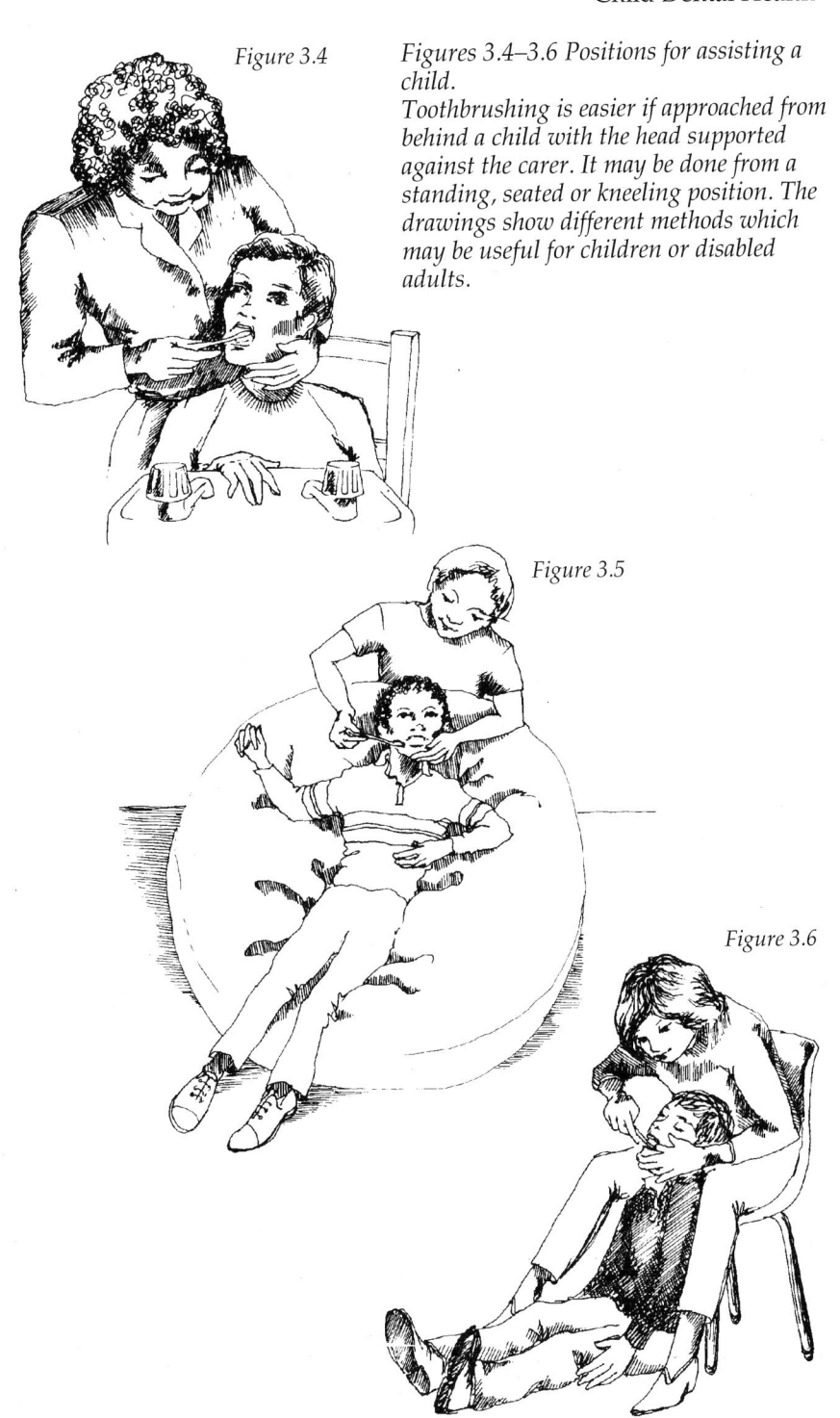

Figure 3.4

Figures 3.4–3.6 Positions for assisting a child.
Toothbrushing is easier if approached from behind a child with the head supported against the carer. It may be done from a standing, seated or kneeling position. The drawings show different methods which may be useful for children or disabled adults.

Figure 3.5

Figure 3.6

For maximum effect, the daily supplement should be in contact with the teeth for as long as possible. Tablets should be sucked or chewed. If the supplement is taken at bedtime after brushing, the length of contact time with the teeth will be even longer. To regulate the total ingestion of fluoride, the amount of fluoridated toothpaste should be restricted to a pea-sized portion on the brush.[23]

All individuals should use fluoridated toothpaste on a daily basis. The decision to use extra supplements in low-fluoridated water areas depends on two major risk factors. The first factor is the individual and social susceptibility to dental caries; this can be either a previous high experience of dental caries in the primary dentition, or a previous high caries experience amongst older siblings.

The second factor is the risk of complications from the effects of chronic illness, dental disease, or dental treatment. This includes medical conditions in which an individual is at risk from bacteraemia, bleeding disorders, or conditions in which there is a reduced ability to combat infection. Learning disabilities or other special needs may produce additional barriers to receiving dental care and emphasise the need for the maximum preventive benefits from fluoride supplements (see Section 3).

The dosages for home-use fluoride supplements are listed in Chapter 2, but will vary depending on the fluoride level in drinking water. This information is available from local dentists or, in the UK, the Dental Public Health Department of the District Health Authority.

Fluoride gels and varnishes can also be applied by a member of the dental team from two to four times a year depending on individual risk.

Regular dental visits
There is a wide variation in how often visits are made to the dentist when the reason is not for pain relief.[24] The factors involved in the decision to attend are a combination of whether there is a perceived need on the part of the individual, or their parent or guardian, and the acceptability and accessibility of the dental service. As a professional group, dentists have had encouraging success in mobilising considerable portions of society to attend regularly or to feel guilty if they do not.[25]

There are a number of clear, research-based, reasons for regular attendance. These include:

- Monitoring the efficiency of plaque removal.
- Early detection of dental caries to ensure a more minimal intervention.
- Early detection of orthodontic problems.
- Screening for other disorders, including malignant and premalignant conditions.

As a baseline, a yearly examination should be the norm[26], but children should be seen more frequently during the stages of dental development.

3.9 Phase 4: Evaluation

A number of health outcome criteria can be used to evaluate the preventive approach, but because dental disease progresses relatively slowly, it can take several years to see results. As most preventive methods are linked to behavioural change, it is possible to monitor effectiveness. These changes could be in dietary practices, improvements in oral hygiene or increased use of dental services.

It is important that observed changes in behaviour are used for evaluation. Unfortunately, the dental profession has often used fear-arousal as a motivating factor, and this has led to the tendency for people to be less open in their accounts of dental health behaviour.

Several indicators of good gingival health can be used to evaluate the effectiveness of oral hygiene measures. These include the absence of bleeding when brushing, as well as the colour and appearance of the gingival tissues (*Colour Plate* **1**).

3.10 Summary

There are clear indications for establishing a thorough preventive regime during childhood, including:

- Attention to the anatomical and developmental aspects of the dentition, so that dental disease and early loss of primary teeth can be avoided.
- Early experience of dental care, if unpleasant and painful, strongly contributes to producing dental anxiety. This will affect dental health beliefs and dental health behaviour in adulthood.

Any preventive strategy should contain four broad phases.

Assessment
This should include the dental health beliefs and behaviour of the parent or guardian and other opinion-formers in the home environment, as this will largely shape the dental health behaviour of the child.

Planning
An holistic approach, which uses preventive approaches incorporated into general nutrition, hygiene and grooming and the use of preventive health services, will be most successful. The approaches will be modified by identifying those individuals with high-risk factors, including medical, physical, mental, social and geographical factors, and past disease experience.

Implementation
Small incremental changes in dietary patterns, oral hygiene techniques, and the use of fluoride will provide a sound basis for the self-caring adult.

Evaluation
Simple, observable changes in behaviour can be used to evaluate success and reinforce the approaches. Changes in actual dental disease can be difficult to monitor due to the need for specialised knowledge and the relatively slow progression of the disease process.

3.11 References

1. Cole, A.G. (1973). The demographic transition. In: *The International Population Conference*. Liège, International Union for Scientific Study of Population, pp. 53–71.
2. World Health Organisation. (1985). *Oral Health Care Systems: An International Collaborative Study*. London, Quintessence, p. 58.
3. World Health Organisation. (1985). *Oral Health Care Systems: An International Collaborative Study*. London, Quintessence, p. 107.
4. Olojugba, O.O. and Lennon, M.A. (1990). Sugar consumption in 5- and 12-year-old school-children in Ondo State, Nigeria, in 1985. *Community Dental Health*, **7**, 259–265.
5. Davis, P. (1987). *Introduction to the Sociology of Dentistry*. Dunedin, New Zealand, Otago Press, p. 58.
6. Davis, P. (1987). Introduction to the Sociology of Dentistry. Dunedin, New Zealand, Otago Press, p. 48–50.
7. Finch, H., Keegan, J., Ward, K. and Sen, B.S. (1988). *Barriers to the Receipt of Dental Care: a qualitative study*. London, Social and Community Planning Research.
8. Murray, J.J. (1987). The potential for prevention in children. In: Elderton, R.J. (Ed.) *Positive Dental Prevention. The Prevention in Childhood of Dental Disease in Adult Life*. Oxford, Heinemann, p. 4.
9. Murray, J.J. (1987). Special considerations in the restoration of deciduous teeth. In: Elderton, R.J. (Ed.) *Positive Dental Prevention. The Prevention in Childhood of Dental Disease in Adult Life*. Oxford, Heinemann, p. 93.
10. Sermel, O. (1974). Emotional and medical factors in child dental anxiety. *J. Child Psychol. Psychiatry*, **15**, 313–321.
11. Davis, P. (1980). *Introduction to the Sociology of Dentistry*. Otago Press, p. 31.
12. Green, L.W. (1970). Should health education abandon change strategies? Perspectives from recent research. *Health Education Monographs*, **30**, 25–47.
13. Pill, R. and Stott, N.C.H. (1985). Choice or change: further evidence on ideas of illness and responsibility for health. *Social Sciences in Medicine*, **20**, 981–90.
14. Hendricks, S.J.H., Freeman, R. and Sheiham, A. (1990). Why inner city mothers take their children for routine medical and dental examinations. *Community Dental Health*, **7**, 33–41.
15. Elderton, R.J. (1987). *Positive Dental Prevention. The Prevention in Childhood of Dental Disease in Adult Life*. Oxford, Heinemann, p. 27.

16. COMA, Department of Health. (1989). *Dietary Sugars and Human Disease. Report of the Panel on Medical Aspects of Food Policy.* Report No. 37. London, HMSO.
17. Traeen, B. and Rise, J. (1990). Dental health behaviours in a Norwegian population. *Community Dental Health*, **7**, 59–68.
18. Hodge, H.C., Holloway, P.J. and Bell, C.R. (1982). Factors associated with toothbrushing behaviour in adolescents. *Br. Dent. J.*, **152**, 49–51.
19. World Health Organisation. (1985). *Oral Health Care Systems. An International Collaborative Study.* London, Quintessence, p. 105.
20. MacGregor, I.D.M. (1987). Toothbrushing frequency in relation to family size and bedtimes in English schoolchildren. *Comm. Dent. Oral Epidemiol.*, **15**, 181–183.
21. Andlaw, R.J. (1987). Fluorides in caries. In: Elderton, R.J. (Ed.) *Positive Dental Prevention. The Prevention in Childhood of Dental Disease in Adult Life.* Oxford, Heinemann, p. 52.
22. Wolfe, W.B., Jackson, D. and James, P.M.C. (1975). Fluoridation in Anglesey: a clinical study. *Br. Dent. J.*, **138**, 165–171.
23. Health Education Authority. (1989). *The Scientific Basis of Dental Health Education.* London, HEA, p. 118.
24. World Health Organisation. (1985). *Oral Health Care Systems. An International Collaborative Study.* London, Quintessence, p. 115.
25. Davis, P. (1987). *Introduction to the Sociology of Dentistry.* Dunedin, New Zealand, Otago Press, p. 91.
26. Health Education Authority. (1989). *The Scientific Basis of Dental Health Education.* London, HEA, p. 14.

4 Oral Care For Older People

4.1 Introduction
4.2 Disability and age
4.3 Oral effects of ageing
4.4 Oral status
4.5 Oral and dental health
4.6 Barriers to dental care
4.7 Routine check-ups
4.8 Oral care
4.9 Summary
4.10 References

4.1 Introduction

General health care is important for all ages. Good oral hygiene is a vital aspect of health care and a comfortable healthy mouth is just as important for older people as for any other section of the population. For older people who may be suffering from illness or disability, maintaining a healthy mouth may play a significant part in the process of rehabilitation and recovery.

Care of the mouth is a necessary part of personal daily care. Primary health care professionals are in a position to encourage older people to take good care of their mouths and to maintain oral health. It is their role to motivate, assist or provide oral care if the individual is dependent as a result of illness or disability. They are therefore in a prime position to identify oral problems which may go unnoticed unless the individual is seeing a dentist regularly.

The mouth and associated structures play an important physiological role in mastication and nutrition. However, the social importance of the mouth in both speech and appearance is often a neglected aspect in older people. A healthy functional mouth has a contribution to make in the process of rehabilitation. The ability to communicate and the dignity and self-esteem given by self-confidence in one's appearance have obvious psychological benefits. Aside from systemic benefits, a nourishing and well-balanced diet contributes to general health and a sense of well-being.

With the onset of illness, deterioration in the individual's ability to manage personal care leads to a cycle of problems associated with neglect, which may cause a change in diet leading to poor nutrition and further physical deterioration. A mouth ulcer, sharp tooth or loose dentures may contribute to, or even precipitate, this change in diet. These are problems which can usually be easily treated if identified at an early stage.

The objective – a comfortable and healthy mouth, which permits a balanced and nutritional diet, looks good and allows communication – is of obvious benefit. To achieve this, it is helpful to have some understanding of the oral and dental problems of older people and the barriers, both real and perceived, which they experience in obtaining dental care.

4.2 Disability and age

In discussing the elderly population and their use of services, the self-evident increase in disability with age must be considered. A recent OPCS survey[1] estimates that 6.2 million of the adult population of Great Britain, of which 4.2 million are aged 60 or more, have a level of disability above that laid down by the criteria for the survey. The survey quite clearly illustrates the prevalence of disability with increasing age.

Among the elderly, the overall rate of disability increases with age, accelerating after 50 years. It rises very steeply after 70 years, with almost 70% of disabled adults being over 60 years, and almost 50% aged 70 or over (*Figure 4.1*). The most severely disabled were reported to be living mainly in residential or institutional care.

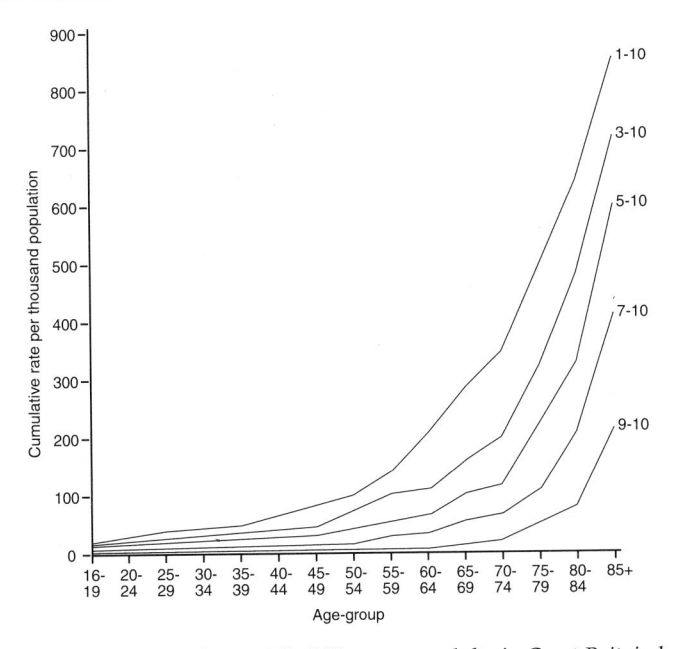

Figure 4.1 Estimates of prevalence of disability among adults in Great Britain by age and severity category. (Reproduced by kind permission of OPCS, Crown copyright).[1]

Mobility was the most frequently reported functional problem with hearing impairment and the inability to manage personal care affecting more than a third of the disabled. Among the elderly disabled, approximately 20% of those aged 60-74 years were estimated to have impaired mobility, rising to 46% in those aged over 75. Most of these elderly disabled people were reported to be living in their own homes, and therefore less easily identifiable except through contact with statutory agencies. The introduction of annual surveillance for over-75s in the new GP contract provides an opportunity to identify and screen for oral problems. A simple questionnaire as a means of alerting health carers to oral and dental problems has been reported.[2]

It has been stressed that caring for the mouth requires a certain level of manual dexterity. Functional disabilities are likely to severely restrict access to dental care and information on services, and will pose limitations on the management of personal oral care. A recent study[3] has confirmed the significant association between the severity of disability and total tooth loss (edentulousness) in the elderly. Eighty per cent of the sample classified as being severely disabled were edentulous, compared with 55% of those categorised as having no disability. Furthermore, those in the severe disability category were more likely to have dentures over 20 years old and were less likely to have seen a dentist in the previous 10 years.[3]

4.3 Oral effects of ageing

Tooth loss is not an inevitable consequence of ageing, although there are changes in oral tissues and surrounding structures which are associated with the ageing process. The degree of change depends on a variety of individual factors:

- Genetic influences.
- Experience of disease.
- Lifestyle.
- Nutrition.
- Habits.

Teeth

The structure of the tooth undergoes a number of changes. Tooth substance is lost through wear; this is called attrition. The degree of wear is related to diet, habits such as grinding the teeth (bruxism), and to the extra load which may be placed on remaining teeth when some teeth have been lost (*Colour Plate* **2**). Attrition of the biting surfaces may lead to a loss of face height, although this is sometimes compensated for by an extra deposit of cement around the roots of the teeth (hypercementosis).

Enamel may also be lost due to erosion (*Colour Plate* **13**; Chapter 2), or abrasion as a result of excessive or incorrect brushing techniques (*Colour*

Plate **14**). Abrasion is most pronounced at the necks of the teeth where the gum may have receded. Enamel also appears to darken with age due to the formation of additional layers of dentine within the tooth. The overall effect is that teeth become less sensitive to external stimuli.

Decay occurs more frequently in the exposed root surface (*Colour Plate* **10**). It is thought to be due to receding gums (gingival recession) exposing dentine which covers the root surface. Dentine, which is less resistant to caries than enamel, together with poor oral hygiene and a soft diet, creates the ideal conditions for root caries – the characteristic pattern of dental caries in the older person.

Changes in structure with age make teeth more brittle. This increases the risk of fracture, particularly when teeth are being extracted. Cementum deposits around the roots may also create complications for extractions. These are important considerations in planning dental treatment.

Bone

Age changes in bone also affect the jaws. Increased porosity of the jaw bones and bone resorption, which follow tooth loss, make jaw bones more brittle. The surface (cortical) bone becomes thinner and, in many older people, the loss of bony ridges leads to difficulty in wearing dentures, particularly in the lower jaw.

Bone previously affected by periodontal disease resorbs more quickly. Loss of function and wearing dentures which are entirely supported by tissue rather than tooth lead to increased bone loss. The changes described predispose to fractures and slower healing, which have implications for dental treatment in the older population, and lead to greater difficulty in the construction of stable dentures.

Oral tissues

Mucous membranes generally atrophy with age. In the mouth, the rate at which this occurs depends on diet, habits, denture wear and oral hygiene. The epithelium covering the cheeks and lips tends to become more keratinised, while the palate becomes less keratinised. Thinner oral mucosa is more easily damaged and penetrated by some substances in food, which may give rise to an itching or burning sensation.

Saliva and salivary glands

There is little evidence to suggest a decrease in salivary flow with ageing, although the composition of saliva appears to have fewer protective properties[4]. Changes in the structure of the salivary glands are recorded. However, medication or disease of the salivary glands may reduce salivary flow, leading to a dry mouth (xerostomia). Thinner oral mucosa and a reduction in saliva lead to problems with eating, speech, swallowing, and the management of dentures.

Summary
Oral changes which may occur as a part of the normal process of ageing or as a result of oral disease may lead to considerable oral discomfort. The immediate effect may be a change in dietary habits with the potential for a reduction in the individual's general health.

4.4 Oral status

Most older people have lost all of their natural teeth but the numbers who are edentulous (with no natural teeth) are gradually declining.[5] This is notable among younger age groups who are themselves approaching retirement (*Tables 4.1, 4.2*).

In the 1988 National Survey of Dental Health[5], 37% of 55–64 year olds had no natural teeth compared to 17% in the 45–54-year-old group. Older people in the unskilled manual groups were much more likely to have lost all their teeth than older people in professional groups.[6] Regional differences were noted, with Scotland and Wales having higher levels of tooth loss than England, and the North of England and Scotland having significantly higher levels than the South of England. More older women have lost all their teeth than men.[6]

The picture of tooth loss appears to be gradually changing as more people are retaining some or all of their natural teeth into later life. It is anticipated that, if the trend continues, future generations of elderly people will be less likely to lose their natural teeth and become edentulous. Furthermore, their expectations of dental health will be greater. In planning dental services for older people, the dental profession anticipates that fewer complete dentures will be needed but more partial dentures, fillings and treatment for gum disease.

4.5 Oral and dental health

Most dental surveys of oral health in the elderly have demonstrated that about three-quarters of the population examined had a need for some form of treatment. Many of these surveys were carried out on specific populations in residential or sheltered accommodation. The results were fairly consistent with national surveys of adult dental health.[7] Treatment needs consisted of:

- Lack of dentures.
- Loose dentures.
- Badly fitting dentures.
- Denture-related conditions.
- Ulcers.
- Decay.
- Gum disease.
- Extractions.

Table 4.1 People with no natural teeth.[5]

Year of survey	Age group (years) 75+	65-74
1968	88%	79%
1985	80%	61%
1988	80%	57%

Table 4.2 People with no natural teeth in 1988 national survey of dental health.[5]

Age group (years)	Percentage with no natural teeth
45-54	17%
55-64	37%
65-74	57%
75+	80%

Approximately a quarter of the sample examined felt they needed treatment and their complaints fell into three main categories:

- Pain and discomfort.
- Difficulty with eating.
- Unacceptable appearance.

The large difference between the dental profession's assessment of need (normative need) and the low perception which older people seem to have of oral problems (subjective need) is a real barrier to older people seeking dental care.

4.6 Barriers to dental care

The apparent low awareness of the need for treatment is not the only barrier to regular dental care in the elderly. Many more have been identified: physical, economic, social and psychological.[7,8] They may be due to past dental experiences and habits, lack of knowledge, inaccurate beliefs, and professional attitudes, as well as much more practical factors, such as cost, transport, illness and restricted mobility.

Mobility

Increasing mobility problems with age restrict access to services. Public transport may be difficult to use, inaccessible, or unavailable. Lack of transport and poor public transport services seriously affect mobility. Dental practices with entrance steps or surgeries on the first floor may be inaccessible. The distance from the nearest dental practice may be relevant in rural areas.

For the frail, disabled and housebound, visiting the dentist may be impossible or, at least, difficult or distressing. This factor is reflected in the way in which low dental attendance is related to the severity of disability[3]; 36% of the housebound, 52% of those needing assistance and 66% of those able to go out without assistance were reported to have seen the dentist in the previous 10 years. Mobility was significantly associated with non-attendance and access was also quoted as a reason for non-attendance.[3]

Economic reasons

The cost of dental treatment is the most commonly quoted reason for not seeing the dentist. In studies of the elderly, few people were aware of the actual cost of treatment, or of exemptions from charges.[9,10] Compared with the cost of seeing a doctor which is currently free under the NHS, it may not be surprising that dental treatment is perceived as expensive by comparison, even though the actual cost may be low.

As well as the cost of dental treatment, the additional expense of transport must be considered.[11] The cost of public transport and/or taxis may be high, particularly in rural areas, and must be viewed in the context of the fall in income which most older people experience on retirement. Understanding the benefits system and keeping up with its changes is almost a full-time occupation. Older people may refuse to apply for benefits to which they may be entitled; this may stem from a feeling of pride or may be simply due to lack of information or confusion on benefits and how to claim them.[9,10]

Those who receive a state pension as their only source of income and those on a low income with no savings are entitled to free dental treatment. The exemption system is more complicated; income from other pensions or savings is taken into consideration, although the ceiling on savings which an individual or couple may hold without penalty has recently been increased. This has raised the threshold for financial assistance for dental treatment and increased the numbers who may be exempt from payment.

Detailed information about the current system for exemptions can be found in DSS leaflet D11, which is regularly updated following legislative changes (Chapter 5). Application for exemption or help with charges involves completing an AG1 (available from DSS offices, opticians, dentists and hospitals), a daunting task in the authors' opinion, although it is understood that this is being revised. If there is any doubt about payment, then individuals should be encouraged to apply for help with charges by completing an AG1A; assistance in completing the application may be required. This is a matter which needs to be handled with sensitivity as an individual's financial status is a personal matter. A recent report by the National Association of Citizens' Advice Bureaux[12] points out the inadequacy and inaccuracy of information and advice given to people by health care staff responsible for operating the scheme.

Fear and anxiety

Older people seem to have a much clearer memory of their youth than of recent events.[13] Previous experiences of dental treatment may have a negative effect. This must be set in the context of experiences of dentistry in its early days when its practice was rather different from today. Off-putting professional attitudes towards older people are referred to in a survey by Age Concern.[14]

Information about dental services
Few older people seem to be aware of the availability of domiciliary dental care or that a home visit is free.[15] Research has highlighted the low levels of awareness of community services which are available, and the importance of ensuring the elderly population is better informed about services.[16]

Beliefs
The belief that teeth are inevitably lost with age seems to be commonly held, even though tooth loss in this age group is probably due to restricted dental services in youth and the practice of extractions and the provision of dentures as the norm. Another commonly held belief is that dentures are the ultimate solution to years of dental pain and that they last for years, in some cases for life[17] (Colour Plate **32**). The practice in some Welsh Valleys of the father paying for extractions and dentures as a wedding present for his daughter is more than anecdotal among general dental practitioners in South Wales; fortunately, this practice now seems to be dying out.

Negative comments such as 'wasting the dentist's time' and not wishing to 'bother the dentist' have been noted.[15,18] It may be that negative attitudes to dental care are associated with negative stereotypes of ageing and repeated experiences of ageism from professionals.[14] Greater awareness in the 'middle-aged' groups, who are more likely to have teeth, are themselves approaching retirement, and are more likely to make demands for services, may eventually result in a reduction in negative beliefs among older people.

Dental attendance
Studies of dental attendance patterns in samples of older people confirm that older people visit the dentist less and less with increasing age. In a survey carried out in North-East England, 30% said they had not visited the dentist for 21 years.[19] In another study, 46% of those aged 65–74 and 63% of those aged over 75 had not visited the dentist for more than 10 years, while 83% of the younger age group and 93% of the older age group had not visited the dentist within the last year.[20] In an area of South Wales, 33% had not seen a dentist for 10 years with significantly fewer dental attendances occurring in the manual group than the non-manual group.[3]

Cultural barriers
A lack of dental care experience in older people who are immigrants from countries with less developed health care systems may contribute towards low attendance in this group.[21] Of this population, 14.9% claimed to attend regularly, with the lack of perceived need being the main reason for non-attendance, unless the subject was in pain or needed new dentures. Barriers relating to language, communication, and a lack of knowledge of cultural beliefs and practices are identified.[22] Although ethnic groups form a culturally diverse and small proportion of the elderly population in the

UK, the danger of overlooking their differing needs and problems are highlighted in the Government White Paper, 'Growing Older'.[23]

Summary
The barriers described give some insight into why older people in the UK tend to visit the dentist less and less frequently with increasing age. However, with regular advice and support from professionals and carers most would benefit. Similar barriers are identified throughout North America and Europe.[24] Sensitivity to the needs of older people and the barriers quoted must be considered in attempting to change the oral health behaviour patterns of this group and ensure appropriate access to dental services.[8]

4.7 Routine check-ups

Regular examination of the mouth is an effective screening method for suspected oral cancers which occur more frequently with increasing age (*Colour Plates* **28, 29, 30**). With early diagnosis, the prognosis is much improved. Long-standing irritation from dentures (*Colour Plate* **31**) which rub, or from a sharp tooth, may increase the risk, and ulcers that persist for more than two weeks should be examined by a dentist.

Potential premalignant conditions can be treated and monitored. This may involve advice on denture use and hygiene, adjusting dentures to prevent irritation, or smoothing a sharp-edged tooth. Counselling on avoiding risk behaviour may be necessary, and information on risk behaviour should be more freely available. Screening is perhaps the most important reason for encouraging annual check-ups in this age group.[25]

An annual dental check-up is recommended as a minimum for all adults, whatever their dental or denture status; this applies to individuals with no natural teeth or dentures. Hard and soft tissues can be examined and dentures checked to ensure they fit well and are not causing soft tissue damage. At the same time, the mouth is screened for oral disease and systemic illnesses which exhibit oral signs or symptoms.

4.8 Oral care

Given the normally high oral and dental needs in the elderly, as shown by various surveys[26], it is very likely that such needs will be found in a health professional's elderly patients or clients. A single question as to whether the patient or client has a dentist, or whether they have seen a dentist in the last year, may be all that is needed to identify those in need.[2]

There will be local variations in the organisation of dental services (Chapter 5) and procedures for referral. The Family Health Services

Authority (formerly the Family Practitioners' Committee) or the Community Dental Service should be contacted for advice on dental services in each district.

The principles and practice of oral care for a self-caring individual apply; care of the teeth, mouth and dentures are described in detail in Chapter 2. Dietary reduction of refined sugars and effective plaque control are essential in the elderly dentate patient, as any reduction in salivary flow increases the risk of dental decay and periodontal disease. A reduction in salivary flow may be exacerbated by xerostomic medication.

When self-care deteriorates, practical advice and assistance will be required. Encouragement may be all that is necessary as a prompt. However, the dependent elderly person who cannot carry out effective oral care techniques will be reliant upon a carer – professional or otherwise – for this personal need.

Practical aspects of oral care

Oral tissues may be thin, inelastic, and more susceptible to damage with increasing age, so care must be taken in providing oral care. A small, soft, multi-tufted toothbrush used gently is advisable.

When providing oral care for a dependent person, the best method is with the individual seated, and the head supported gently against the body for all techniques, whether toothbrushing, towelling or swabbing (*Figure 4.2*). It is more difficult to perform oral care for the bedfast individual, unless the individual is sitting up. Oral care for the dependent and dysphagic (swallowing difficulties) is described in Chapter 16.

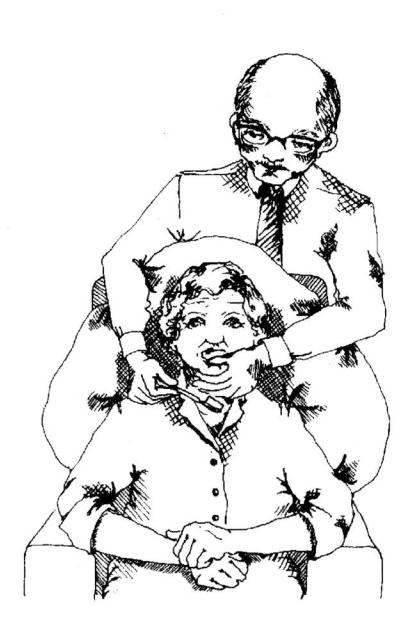

Figure 4.2 Providing oral care for an older person.

If toothbrushing is difficult, then teeth can be towelled with a piece of gauze soaked in chlorhexidine gluconate gel or mouthwash and wrapped around a gloved finger. This will help to control plaque, and this method can also be used to sweep away food debris and cleanse soft tissues.

Chemical plaque control

The bacterial content of plaque can be effectively reduced by chlorhexidine gluconate (Chapters 2, 9 and 16). This may be used as an adjunct to toothbrushing and to reduce plaque on dentures. It is particularly useful for those who are more at risk of oral and dental disease due to medical or behavioural problems, or when toothbrushing is difficult due to poor co-operation.

Mouth care

Most people who have lost their natural teeth wear dentures. Dentures facilitate chewing and help to maintain a normal diet, and thus good nutrition, digestion, and elimination. The choice of wearing dentures is, of course, up to the individual, and many people seem to manage to eat quite well with only one denture or no dentures. The success of any treatment to construct new dentures depends largely upon the individual's motivation. If the individual is able to eat adequately and does not want dentures, then his or her decision should be respected, although counselling and advice may sometimes help them to see the benefits.

Whether or not dentures are worn, the mouth still needs to be cleaned. The mouth should be rinsed after meals to remove food debris. Gums and palate should be brushed with a small soft toothbrush. If mouth-washing or brushing cannot be tolerated, then all surfaces of the mouth should be wiped with gauze using a sweeping action to remove food debris. Food tends to pouch in the folds between the gums and cheeks, so attention should be paid to these areas. Even if there is limited co-operation for oral care, it is usually possible to cleanse areas between the gums and cheeks using a gentle sweeping action.

Care of dentures

This has been covered quite comprehensively in Chapter 2. If the patient or client insists on wearing dentures at night, both mouth and dentures must be scrupulously clean. The importance of removing dentures at night cannot be stressed too often. Night-time denture wearers are prone to develop a condition sometimes called 'denture sore mouth'. This is a misnomer; it is usually caused by candidal infection (Chapter 14) of the soft tissue areas in contact with the denture, due to plaque and poor denture hygiene (*Colour Plates* **22, 23**).

Dentures, just like natural teeth, become coated with food and plaque. Plaque is not easily visible, until quite a thick deposit has formed over a number of days. Hard deposits may form in this layer to produce tartar (calculus). This makes the denture rough and unhygienic and may cause irritation; the wearer may be unaware of the slowly accumulating deposit. The points to remember about denture care are:

- Remove after meals.
- Brush with a tooth or denture brush.
- Use ordinary unperfumed household soap.
- Clean over a basin of cold water.
- Rinse well before replacing in the cleaned mouth.
- To remove hard deposits, refer to dentist.

It is also important to note *soaking alone does not remove plaque*. This is only removed effectively by brushing.

Other points to remember in regularly handling a patient's or client's dentures are:

- Check for rough or sharp areas.
- Check for hard deposits.
- Check whether denture is labelled.
- Refer to dentist if necessary.

Dentures that are dirty, old or worn may damage delicate oral tissues, and lead to conditions such as ulcers, soreness and infection. Chronic denture inflammation may lead to potentially premalignant oral pathology (*Colour Plate* 31). If any area of soreness or ulceration appears and persists (*Colour Plate* 30), the advice of a dentist should be obtained.

A cycle of problems with dentures is associated with illness in the elderly. Initially, the individual may have a reduced ability to cope with dentures or a reduced tolerance to wearing dentures. Oral and denture hygiene may be neglected and increasingly the dentures are not worn, leading to poor nutrition and further physical deterioration. A dental opinion should be requested.

Dentures that have been worn for many years are usually very acceptable to the wearer, rather like a comfortable pair of old slippers, even though teeth may have worn and bony ridges shrunk so much that dentures no longer fit. Over the years, the older person acclimatises to the changes and may be unaware that the dentures no longer fit. These problems are often identified following a stroke when facial paralysis may lead to an inability to control dentures.

Minor adjustments to improve the fit by inserting a temporary or permanent soft lining are relatively simple and effective procedures. If changes are well-tolerated, then old dentures can be copied, eliminating the bad features but retaining the general shape. This is often the best method of improving existing dentures, or of providing new dentures for people who have acclimatised to their old worn ones. Constructing new dentures for a patient who may be unable to co-operate, or who lacks motivation, is difficult and at times impossible. However, the effect of facial paralysis can be modified by enlarging dentures on the affected side, restoring facial contour and reducing the tendency to drool (Chapter 10).

Naming dentures

Newer dentures may be marked with the owner's name. As this is a fairly recent practice, many older dentures are not named. Admission to hospital or residential care is often accompanied by confusion and disorientation, and dentures may be lost or misplaced. Fortunately, the misguided practice of cleaning all dentures together in a large bowl, which the authors have encountered, is rare. In such a case, it can be difficult or impossible, even for a dentist, to identify the correct owner of dentures.

Naming dentures is a sensible practice. It does not prevent denture loss, but if found dentures can be identified and returned to the owner. New dentures can be labelled in construction, and the dental practice may provide this service. Naming takes a few minutes, and it is recommended that this is carried out on admission to hospital or residential care, with the individual or family's agreement. A denture-marking kit, which can also be used to name spectacles, is described in Chapter 2.

Toothbrushing aids

Simple aids to help people who may have difficulty in gripping a tooth or denture-brush, or who may have lost the use of one hand, are described in detail in Chapter 9. Simple adaptations include increasing the width of the handle by various means, bending the handle or lengthening it, or attaching a device such as a palm strap. The dentist, hygienist or occupational therapist will be able to advise.

4.9 Summary

Dental conditions handicap the elderly.[27] Improving the oral and dental health of the older generation is a major objective of the dental profession.[25] Much need has been identified in various studies. The development of dental services which are tailored to the needs of the individual must address the barriers which have been described. Identification of the elderly, frail, and housebound, can only be achieved by an 'out-reach' approach in liaison with health, statutory and voluntary agencies who care for the elderly.

By providing information on the dental needs of the elderly, the availability of dental services and the principles and practice of good oral care, it is anticipated that primary health care professionals will be better equipped to identify problems, care for the oral needs of the older generation and access dental services.

4.10 References

1. Martin, J., Meltzer, H. and Elliot, D. (1988). *The Prevalence of Disability Among Adults: Report 1.* London, OPCS, Social Survey Division, HMSO.
2. Hoad-Reddick, G. (1991). A study to determine oral health needs of institutionalised elderly patients by non-dental health care workers. *Comm. Dent. Oral Epidemiol.*, **19**, 233–236.
3. Jones, D. and Lester, C. (1993). *Dental health of a random community-based elderly population.* Research Team, Department of Geriatric Medicine, UWCM, Cardiff.
4. Flint, S. and Scully, C. (1988). Orofacial age changes and related diseases. *Dental Update*, Oct., 337–342.
5. Adult Dental Health 1988. (1990). *Br. Dent. J.*, April 7, 279–281.
6. Downer, M.C. (1991). The Improving Dental Health of United Kingdom Adults and Prospects for the Future. *Br. Dent. J.*, Feb 23, 154–158.
7. Clerehugh, A. (1986). Dental services for handicapped elderly people. A British Association for the Study of Community Dentistry Policy Document. *Community Dental Health*, **3**, 175–181.
8. Griffiths, J.E. (1991). The dental needs of the elderly and the delivery of care. In: Pathy, M.S.J. *Principles and Practice of Geriatric Medicine.* Bristol, John Wiley, p. 356–358.
9. Manderson, R.D. and Ettinger, R.L. (1975). Dental status of institutionalised elderly population of Edinburgh. *Comm. Dent. Oral. Epidemiol.*, **3**(3), 100–107.
10. Schou, L. and Eadie, D. (1991). Qualitative study of oral health norms and behaviour among elderly people in Scotland. *Community Dental Health*, **8**, 53–58.
11. Kail, B.I.P. and Silver, M.M. (1984). Dental demands of elderly people living at home in Hampshire. *Br. Dent. J.*, **157**(3), 94–97.
12. National Association of Citizens Advice Bureaux. (1991). *Health Warning: Low Income Groups and Health Benefits.* London, NACAB.
13. Finch, H., Keegan, J., Ward, K. and Sen, B.S. (1988). Barriers to the receipt of dental care. A qualitative research study. *Social and Community Planning Research*, p.35.
14. Age Concern. (1982). *Towards Better Dental Health for Elderly People.* London, Age Concern.
15. Smith, J.C. and Sheiham, A. (1980). Dental treatment needs and demands of an elderly population in England. *Comm. Dent. Oral Epidemiol.*, **8**(7), 360–364.
16. Salvage, A.V., Jones, D. and Vetter, N.J. (1988). Awareness of and satisfaction with community services in a random sample of over-75s. *Health Trends*, **20**, 88–92.
17. Ritchie, G.M. and Simpson, P.R. (1981). *A Community Study to Examine Attitudes Towards Better Dental Health and the Demand and Need for Dental Care.* London, University College, University of London.
18. Osborne, J., Maddick, I., Gould, A. and Ward, D. (1979). Dental demands of old people in Hampshire. *Br. Dent. J.*, **146**(11), 351–355.
19. Hoad-Reddick, G., Grant, A.A. and Griffiths, C.S. (1987). The dental health of an elderly population in north-west England: results of a survey undertaken in Halton Health Authority. *J. Dent.*, **15**(4), 139–146.
20. Broadway, E.S. and Kemp, F.M. (1985). Dental attendance of elderly people in East Anglia. *Br. Dent. J.*, **159**(6), 189-190.
21. Mattin, D. and Smith, J.M. (1991). The oral health status, dental needs and factors affecting utilisation of dental services in Asians aged 55 years and over resident in Southampton. *Br. Dent. J.*, **170**, 369–372.

22. Williams, S.A., Ahmed, I.A. and Hussain, P. (1991). Ethnicity, health and dental care – perspectives among British Asians: 2. *Dental Update*, June, 205–207.
23. Department of Health and Social Security. (1981). *Growing Older*. Cmnd 8173. London, HMSO.
24. Kandelman, D. *et al.* (1986). Dental needs of the elderly: a comparison between some European and North American surveys. *Community Dental Health*, **3**, 19–39.
25. British Dental Association. (1992). *Quality Care for Oral Health*. London, BDA.
26. Griffiths, J.E. 1991. The dental needs of the elderly and the delivery of care. In: Pathy, M.S.J. *Principles and Practice of Geriatric Medicine*. Bristol, John Wiley, p. 354.
27. Smith, J. and Sheiham, A. (1979). How dental conditions handicap the elderly. *Comm. Dent. Oral Epidemiol.*, **7**, 305–310.

5 Dental Services and the Dental Team

5.1 Introduction
5.2 The history of dentistry
5.3 Dental services
5.4 General dental services
5.5 Community dental services
5.6 Hospital dental services
5.7 Domiciliary dental care
5.8 The dental team
5.9 Future developments in dental services
5.10 Summary
5.11 References

5.1 Introduction

The organisation and availability of dental services varies considerably worldwide. The type of service available, whether private fee-paying or state subsidised, depends largely upon the prevailing political philosophy, the country's economic status, the levels of oral and dental disease, and the value placed upon health care systems, particularly upon oral health.

In the UK, the public's perception of dental services seems to be of the dentist 'in private practice' and the 'dental hospital service', with perhaps some knowledge of particular specialist services, such as oral surgery or orthodontics. Changes in the structure of the NHS take time to filter through, not only to the public but also to primary health care professionals, as demonstrated by a survey of the knowledge of general medical practitioners.[1] This section will provide information on the organisation and function of dental services, and the roles of members of the dental team in the UK. Private dental services are beyond the scope of this chapter.

5.2 The history of dentistry

Oral and dental disease has been documented by archaeological studies of the earliest human remains. Evidence of treatment is prehistoric, with the earliest records dating from Egyptian civilisation around 4000 BC.

Quite complex treatment was performed in India from 3000 BC. This included extractions, scaling and gingival surgery, and even the transplantation of animal teeth. Diseased teeth and gums were treated by herbs and acupuncture by the Chinese as early as 2000 BC and extractions are credited to Aesculapius in Greek civilisation in the second century BC. Dentures and bridges made of gold and wired to the teeth were worn by the Etruscans around 700 BC.

Hippocrates wrote of health and dental problems around 460 BC. His writings formed the basis of the Hippocratic oath to which both doctors and, until recently, dentists pledged themselves upon qualification. Following World War Two and as a result of war crimes against certain races and other groups, a revised code of conduct termed the 'Declaration of Geneva' was introduced to unite members of the medical professions worldwide and to introduce an international code of ethics.[2] This is worth quoting, although a longer declaration now forms the 'International Principles of Ethics for the Dental Profession'.

'The Declaration of Geneva'
'At the time of being admitted as a member of the Medical Profession, I solemnly pledge myself to consecrate my life to the service of humanity.

I will give to my teachers the respect and gratitude which is their due.

I will practise my profession with conscience and dignity.

The health of my patient will be my first consideration.

I will respect the secrets which are confided in me.

I will maintain by all the means in my power the honour and the noble traditions of the medical profession.

My colleagues will be my brothers.

I will not permit considerations of religion, nationality, race, party politics or social standing to intervene between my duty and my patient.

I will maintain the utmost respect for human life from the time of conception: even under threat, I will not use my medical knowledge contrary to the laws of humanity.

I make these promises solemnly, freely and upon my honour.'

By the fourth century, extraction and scaling instruments were available, and although there was some scientific knowledge, dentistry was still surrounded by myth and folklore. Healing was traditionally carried out by clergymen until the 12th century, when the Pope banned the clergy from carrying out operations which involved 'blood-letting'. Tooth-drawing then moved into the hands of barbers, barber-surgeons, charlatans and even blacksmiths, and was practised in fairs, markets and even on street corners.

Modern dentistry has its origins in the 18th century when Pierre Fouchard, The Surgeon Dentist to Louis XIV, elevated dentistry to a scientific profession. The birth of the dental profession in the UK took place with the passing of the 1858 Medical Act; this was followed by the first Dental Act of 1878. It was not until the 1921 Dental Act was passed that dentistry

Dental Services and the Dental Team

became a closed profession, and it was only with the advent of the NHS in 1948 that dentistry became freely available to the entire population. Compared with many professions, this makes dentistry a relatively new profession.

5.3 Dental services

Since 1948 there have been many organisational changes in dental services in response to the changing patterns of oral and dental disease and to the socio-political climate. To find the most appropriate dental service, a brief explanation of the roles and functions of each service is necessary. In the UK there are currently three principal dental services available under the NHS:

- General Dental Services.
- Community Dental Services.
- Hospital Dental Services.

5.4 General Dental Services

Most NHS dental care and treatment is provided by general dental practitioners. This is the first choice for routine dental care for most of the population, and a very wide range of preventive and treatment services are available.

All general dental practitioners practising under the NHS are under contract to the Family Health Services Authority (FHSA), previously the district Family Practitioner Committee. In Scotland, this function is carried out by the Health Board and in Northern Ireland by the Central Services Agency. The FHSA or its equivalent, which acts as a mediator between the dentist and the public, holds dental lists for each district. These include some basic practice information. Lists are also held at main post offices, libraries and many other public places, and can also be found in British Telecom's *Yellow Pages*.

Continuing care
Changes in contracts for general dental practitioners took place in 1990, and patients may now register with a dentist for continuing care in the same way as with a family doctor.[3] Under the new contract, a far greater emphasis is placed on preventive care and the involvement of the patient in their treatment plan. Registration under continuing care confers certain other benefits:

- A plan of treatment showing the cost of each item.
- Emergency out-of-hours telephone advice and treatment, if required, normally within 24 hours.
- Free replacement of crowns or fillings less than a year old in certain circumstances.

Since the new system was implemented, minor changes in the regulations governing the provision of treatment plans have reduced the heavy administrative burden on dental practitioners.

The continuing care system for adults lapses if the patient does not attend for two years and for children after one year. It can be discontinued by the patient and ends automatically if the patient registers with another dentist, although it is recommended that the patient advises their previous dentist of the transfer.

This arrangement can also be ended by the dentist:

- By giving three months' notice to the patient and to the FHSA and after completing any current treatment.
- If the dentist–patient relationship appears to have broken down, then the FHSA decides whether to authorise the withdrawal.
- By not renewing the contract at the end of two years, if the patient still owes treatment fees.

If the practice is unable through lack of facilities or expertise to provide the treatment required, the patient may be referred to another practice for continuing care, or for specific parts of the treatment plan, e.g. orthodontic treatment. Some practices specialise in providing only orthodontic treatment. Referrals may also be made to the Community Dental Service or the Hospital Dental Service. The district FHSA, or its equivalent, will advise on local procedures.

The occasional patient

For patients who do not wish to register, treatment can be provided as an 'occasional patient', but the benefits of continuing care do not apply. Occasional patients are not entitled to the full range of NHS treatments and do not have the same rights as those registering for continuing care. The benefits provided by continuing care make it worthwhile registering with a dentist.

Details of the new system are described in a booklet.[3] The district FHSA can provide more detailed and up-to-date advice and information.

Practice information

From October 1991, dentists in general dental practice are required to produce practice information leaflets describing the services provided. These will include information on:

- Normal surgery hours.
- Emergency arrangements.
- Dentists' qualifications and when these were obtained.
- Access to premises without the use of stairs.
- Access for wheelchair users to premises and surgery.
- Disabled toilet facilities.
- Arrangements for home visits.
- In some cases, languages spoken by staff.

Dental Services and the Dental Team

Practice specialities will be described, enabling the public to make a more informed choice in selecting a dentist suitable for their needs. Information on domiciliary dental care is invaluable for people who are frail, disabled or housebound, and although there is no charge for the home visit, NHS charges apply for treatment provided.

Private and NHS treatment

Most practices provide a full range of NHS treatment to rehabilitate the mouth. The new system of continuing care stresses the importance of prevention, particularly for children (Chapter 3) and at-risk groups (Section 3).

Advances in dental techniques and materials now provide a much wider range of restorative and preventive treatments. However, some types of treatment can be carried out only with the prior approval of the Dental Practice Board. The choice of a more expensive form of treatment may also require prior approval. If this is refused, the patient can appeal to the FHSA against the decision.

It is a matter of choice and agreement between the patient and dentist if some or all of the treatment is to be provided privately. Private treatment can be offered as an alternative to NHS, or in addition to it. The treatment plan provides a summary of the treatment agreed. It identifies those items being provided under the NHS and those being provided privately. A patient registered for continuing care signs the treatment plan agreeing to the prescribed treatment and the arrangements made for NHS and any private treatment.

Charges

In 1948 dental treatment under the NHS was free for everyone. Charges have been introduced over the years, the scale of NHS charges being controlled by government legislation. There is evidence that charges deter patients from seeking treatment.[4] The effect of a charge for an examination which was implemented in 1989 has yet to be fully evaluated in terms of dental attendance. The effect of an examination charge for those individuals who are only seeking advice is seen as a negative barrier[4], particularly for those groups who tend to attend only for the relief of pain.

The information provided is based on the most recent legislation. However, the reader should obtain updated information on charges from the FHSA or from a dentist in general dental practice. Certain items of treatment under the NHS are currently free to everyone:

- The arrest of haemorrhage.
- Re-cementing a bridge.
- Repairs to dentures.
- An emergency dental call-out or a home visit.

NHS dental treatment is automatically free for the following groups:

- Children up to their 18th birthday.
- Students in full-time education up to their 19th birthday.

- Expectant women and mothers with a baby under a year old.
- People on Income Support or Family Credit and their spouse or 'partner'.
- Holders of an AG2 certificate.

The patient should notify the dentist of the receipt of Family Credit or Income Support and sign the dental payment form accordingly; in this case, a certificate showing exemption is not required. People who do not fall into these categories but who are, or feel they are, on a low income, should apply for help with the cost of dental charges on form AG1, obtainable from DSS offices, opticians, dentists and hospitals. A detailed account of the system for exemption and the ceiling for savings can be found in the DSS leaflet D11, which is regularly updated following changes in government legislation.

The DSS will advise on the outcome of the application and, if eligible, provide a certificate which is valid for six months. An AG2 certificate entitles the holder to free dental treatment, while an AG3 certificate provides the holder with limited help with the cost of dental charges. As the certificate only lasts six months and confers other benefits, it is worth applying in advance and then every six months thereafter if appropriate.

For patients eligible for payment for NHS treatment, the current charge is 80% of the cost of treatment up to a maximum of £250. This includes examination, X-rays, fillings, crowns, bridges, dentures and all other agreed NHS treatment to maintain the patient's oral health.

The role of the FHSA

The FHSA replaced the Family Practitioners Committee in 1990 as a result of the White Paper, *Promoting better health*[5] and the NHS and Community Care Act.[6] It is responsible for managing and planning family health services in each district; this includes family doctors, dentists, pharmacists and opticians, who are contracted to provide NHS care. The FHSA has a distinctive role to play in liaising with all branches of the health services, with Social Services and the voluntary sector to monitor health, and to promote health and prevention. Further changes are likely to take place in the role of the FHSA by the time this book is in print.

In terms of General Dental Services, the FHSA monitors the new system for continuing dental care and deals with the public's problems in obtaining dental services.

Overview

The system of continuing care is a new concept for General Dental Services under the NHS. It aims to encourage a partnership between the patient and dentist, to encourage regular dental attendance, to maintain oral health, and to prevent future oral or dental disease. It places the responsibility for oral health upon the individual, parent or guardian, with the dentist and dental team providing support to achieve oral health.

While most general dental practitioners in the UK provide the full range of dental care and refer mainly for consultant-based services, there has been a growth in the specialised practice providing only certain types of treatment. The most common in the UK is the orthodontic practice, but there has been an increase in practices providing advanced cosmetic and restorative work. In the USA, it is not uncommon for practices to specialise even as far as particular types of treatment like endodontics (see Glossary). Trends towards more specialised practices will continue as modern dentistry becomes increasingly sophisticated; the full range of expertise and equipment required will encourage practitioners to concentrate on particular areas.

5.5 Community Dental Services

The Community Dental Service emerged from the School Dental Service. The latter was inspired in the early 20th century by a liberal philosophy to 'educate, nourish and provide health care, including dental for the semi-literate and poorly-fed broad mass of English children'.[7] It played a major role in taking dental services to children and the most needy, and followed the principles of dental public health in epidemiology and screening for dental disease.

Legislation in 1978 provided new guidelines for the Community Dental Service on the inclusion of dental services for the elderly or disabled people.[8] The development of these services was left to the discretion of health authorities, provided that their obligations to children were met. In 1987, the White Paper, *Promoting Better Health*[5], offered further guidance on the development of the Community Dental Service with a clear remit to develop dental services for adults with a 'special need'. It provided the Service with a commitment to:

- Monitor levels of dental health in all sections of society.
- Identify those with special needs.
- Organise and provide dental health education.
- Provide a safety net for treatment for those whose needs cannot be met by General Dental Services.

In practical terms, the Community Dental Service complements the General Dental Service in providing dental services to people who are unable to obtain treatment from the latter. The following groups of people are those most likely to receive treatment from the Community Dental Service:

- Those with learning disabilities.
- Those with a physical disability.
- Those suffering mental illness.
- Medically compromised.
- Emotionally handicapped.
- Socially disadvantaged.
- Geographically isolated.

- With communication difficulties.
- Frail, disabled elderly.

The Act[5] offered the opportunity to identify needs, initiate new programmes and to expand existing programmes for delivering dental care to 'special needs' groups in liaison with the General Dental Services. In practical terms, this means that the health professional, carer or the individuals themselves should be able to gain access to appropriate dental services for their particular needs.

Although regular dental care may seem a low priority for many people with a special need, there are several advantages in establishing regular dental contact as opposed to dealing with emergencies. Early contact with the dental team will enable regular screening to be carried out and the development of preventive approaches most appropriate to an individual's needs.

Some people will require dental services from a specialist centre, so an additional layer of referral may be necessary. The Community Dental Service is well-placed to co-ordinate referring patients to dental services according to their needs. It will increasingly develop its out-reach approach in liaison with statutory and voluntary agencies. Aside from more formal contacts, an easily contactable free source of dental advice will prove valuable for daily oral care.

5.6 Hospital Dental Services

The development of Hospital Dental Services centred around the great seats of medical science in the 19th century. Lectures on dental surgery were given at Guy's Hospital in 1799, while in the following year the Royal College of Surgeons received a Royal Charter. Throughout the 19th century dental schools were established, and the first examination in dental surgery was held by the Royal College of Surgeons in 1860. Today, Hospital Dental Services are widely available and organised into three distinct areas:

- Dental teaching hospitals.
- Oral, dental and maxillofacial surgery in general hospitals.
- Oral or dental services to patients in hospital, particularly those in continuing care.

Dental teaching hospitals

The main responsibility of the teaching hospital or dental school is to train future members of the dental profession and ancillary members of the dental team. Teaching hospitals currently remain part of the university academic system. However, consultants in different dental specialities are employed by the NHS primarily to provide specialist services to the public, although teaching is usually included in their contracts.

Training for dental undergraduates is intense and highly specialised. It encompasses a wide range of topics, including general medicine and surgery, behavioural science, epidemiology and community dental health, as well as the range of complex practical skills required to practise modern dental techniques. Courses last five years with a postgraduate vocational training period in one of the three dental services.

Dental therapists, dental hygienists, dental nurses and dental technicians may also be trained. Their roles in the dental team are described later in this chapter.

Hospital Dental Services

Before the Second World War, dental care in provincial hospitals was mainly confined to the extraction of teeth for individuals who were unable to afford dental care. During the War itself, maxillofacial surgery units consisting of a dental surgeon and an anaesthetist were set up mainly in military hospitals. These units spread to civilian hospitals, later to be led by the new consultant grade developed as a result of the 1946 Health Act.

Other consultant specialities appeared, e.g. orthodontics, child dental health and more recently in restorative dentistry, oral medicine and forensic dentistry. Today, teams in these specialities operating under the direction of a consultant will be based in either a dental or medical school, in maxillofacial surgery units, or in district general hospitals.

Referrals for specialist treatment are made mainly by the medical and dental professions, although some hospitals may have a casualty department that treats dental emergencies in the general public.

Dental services to in-patients

Dental services to hospital in-patients are also provided by the Hospital Dental Services and in some districts by the Community Dental Service. This service began in 1976 as a response to the lack of organised dental services to patients in continuing care. Comprehensive routine dental care and annual screening is recommended for patients in hospital for more than 30 days, while emergency dental care is available to all in-patients.

Patients whose illness, injury or treatment puts them more at risk of oral and dental disease, may also require dental services and specific advice on oral care and prevention as part of the process of rehabilitation, e.g. rehabilitation medicine, oncology, cardiology.

Increasingly, staff employed in the Hospital Dental Services are involved in training programmes for general nurses in oral and dental disease, and in establishing nursing standards for oral care. Treatment may be provided in a dental surgery or on the ward, whichever is most appropriate for the individual. There is considerable variation in dental surgery facilities in hospitals providing continuing care. The control of cross-infection poses major practical difficulties for invasive bedside treatment due to resistant micro-organisms.

5.7 Domiciliary dental care

General Dental Service
The dental profession has been carrying out domiciliary care for many years, but health care professionals and the general public seem unaware that this type of care is available. Details of dental practitioners providing domiciliary dental services can be obtained from the FHSA.

When treatment is provided by a general dental practitioner, the visit is free but the usual charges for treatment provided apply. Complex treatment requires sophisticated portable dental equipment which may be too expensive to be held by many general dental practices. However, simple treatment for the relief of pain, preventive care, simple extractions and dentures can be provided with minimal equipment of the type normally held in any general dental practice.

Community Dental Service
The Community Dental Service also provides domiciliary dental care and, in most districts, portable equipment enabling more complex treatment is available. There are also mobile self-drive dental surgeries. These can be driven to the home if complex treatment is required, a service which may sometimes be appropriate for group homes or residential homes, and in areas where there is a shortage of accessible dental practices.

Dental therapists and dental hygienists in the Community Dental Service have an important role in the maintenance of oral health and in giving preventive advice and treatment to people who are housebound, disabled or dependent for oral care.

Referrals are taken from the medical and dental profession, primary health care workers, statutory and voluntary agencies, and in many districts from the individual. The Community Dental Service may also co-ordinate domiciliary dental services for people who are frail, disabled or housebound and ensure that services are available to people who are unable to obtain treatment from the General Dental Service.

5.8 The dental team

Dentistry has become a specialised profession and the trained auxiliary grades which have emerged in recent years make a significant contribution to the team approach to treatment. A brief explanation of the specialities and the roles of auxiliary members of the team is essential.

Dental therapist
Training for dental therapists in the UK began in 1960 at New Cross Hospital, London, but is now undertaken only at the London Hospital.

Dental Services and the Dental Team

Therapists are trained to provide simple dental treatment, particularly for children, and to work in the Hospital and Community Dental Service. Treatment is provided under the written prescription of a dentist and consists of:

- Extracting primary teeth.
- Simple dental fillings.
- Cleaning and polishing teeth.
- Scaling teeth to remove calculus and other debris.
- Application of certain medicaments.
- Application of fluoride and other preventive substances.

Dental hygienist

The first training programmes for dental hygienists started in 1913 in the USA against opposition from many members of the dental profession. Their professional role at the time was described as preventing dental disease. Training in the UK began in the Armed Forces in 1943, heralding a team approach to oral health.

The civilian training programme was preceded by an experimental course at the Eastman Hospital in 1950, and by 1959 the definitive training of dental hygienists began. The General Dental Council laid down strict regulations concerning the role and function of a dental hygienist and the training syllabus. Dental hygienists are now trained in all dental schools in the UK, except in Belfast where training will start in 1993.

A dental hygienist works under the written direction of a registered dental surgeon who has examined the patient and indicated the course of treatment to be provided. This may include:

- Cleaning and polishing.
- Scaling teeth to remove calculus and other debris.
- Application of certain medicaments.
- Application of fluoride and other preventive substances.

Both dental hygienists and therapists are trained in communicating with individuals and groups. They play an important role in individual tuition and group oral health education, and in getting over the basic messages for promoting oral health.

Dental surgery assistant

The dental surgery assistant is perhaps the most familiar member of the dental team. The primary role of the 'dental nurse' is to provide support for the clinical members of the team. This includes the preparation of instruments and materials, and attending to the patient's needs.

Training may be provided within General Dental Practice, the Community Dental Service or in dental teaching hospitals. The nationally approved qualification may also be obtained at Colleges of Further Education and on government training schemes.

The dental surgery assistant is an important link between the individual and the dental service. They are usually skilled communicators who may extend their role to that of dental health educator. A certificate in oral health education is the next step in this direction.

In some countries, the dental surgery assistant may have a limited clinical role, including the placement of filling materials.

Dental health educator

In the more prevention-oriented team, there may be a cadre with the particular role of dental health educator. They often have a dental nurse or dental hygienist background, but may also have primary training in other fields of the caring profession. Their main role is the provision of dental health education programmes to individuals or to small groups. In the UK, Community Dental Services may have dental health promoters working with other education and health professionals who also have a health education role.

Dental technician

The role of the dental technician in replacing missing teeth or tissue with prostheses for functional and cosmetic reasons has become increasingly technical. The prostheses may be dentures, crowns, bridges, implants or designed to replace tissue lost during maxillofacial surgery. New techniques and materials have created the need for greater technical skills.

Even though they are not always visible in the clinical setting, the dental technician is an integral member of the team, who constructs both functional and cosmetic appliances. Historically, the dental technician has been seen as the 'back room boy'. However, many dental technicians are female and, within the team approach, they may be asked to see a patient by the clinician to advise on cosmetic or technical problems.

Training is usually obtained through a general dental practice laboratory, a commercial laboratory, or a hospital dental department linked with day-release to a college. Some colleges offer three-year full-time courses in dental technology.

5.9 Future developments in dental services

A number of factors will affect the way that dental services are carried out in the next decade, not least the prevailing socio-political ideology. As with any health care system, the way the service is financed will determine patterns of care. This, coupled with rising consumerism and more informed dentally aware clients, will place more demands on services. This should encourage more flexible patterns of dental care in terms of when and where it is carried out. Increased use of dental auxiliaries will

Dental Services and the Dental Team

mean that the traditional arrangement of dentist and chairside assistant will gradually disappear and the patient of the future may be treated by a variety of clinical operators.

New technological developments, particularly in the field of dental materials, will drastically alter the way dentistry is carried out. Adhesive, tooth-coloured materials, providing more aesthetic restorations, will require less tooth preparation.

As yet, the use of laser technology in dentistry is in its infancy, but it appears very promising. Soft lasers are being used to speed up healing after surgery, and hard lasers to cut hard tooth substance instead of dental handpieces. One major advantage is in this approach is that it is said not to require local anaesthesia.

Control of pain and discomfort during dental procedures is also undergoing radical change. 'Fear of the needle' is undoubtedly a major barrier to seeking dental care, even though the use of topical anaesthesia, modern fine-bore needles and good technique can reduce the discomfort. A new approach using an electrical field to block transmissions of pain may replace the chemical local anaesthetic in some cases.

Much anxiety and fear of dental treatment can be dealt with effectively by an operator skilled in the techniques of behavioural science, such as behavioural modification, modelling, hypnosis and counselling techniques. Most experienced operators acquire some of these skills through experience and post-qualification training. Such techniques are now receiving a greater prominence in undergraduate training in the UK.

Even when tooth loss has occurred, wearing dentures is not inevitable. In addition to new techniques in fixed bridge work (Chapter 2), the science of implantology is developing fast. This involves surgically inserting 'artificial roots' into the jaw bones to which crowns, bridges, complete or partial dentures can be attached. Although implantology is still very new, there have been major advances in reducing the body's rejection of implants.

Many advances in the treatment of periodontal disease have taken place due to greater understanding of the disease process and the use of new materials which encourage regeneration of some of the lost periodontal tissue.

Even though there has been an overall reduction, the level of dental caries still poses a considerable health problem. Research is continuing into the development of a vaccine against the bacteria in dental plaque which cause caries.

In summary, dental surgery and the range of treatments on offer will change radically over the next decade, coupled with a more preventive approach to oral and dental care. This should make the dental visit a much less stressful and more comfortable experience.

5.10 Summary

Although there are variations between countries in the delivery of services and in the roles of the respective members of the dental team, it is useful for the health professional or carer to have a working knowledge of the dental services. This will facilitate contact between the individual with special needs and the most appropriate sector, as recommended in the dental profession's targets for oral health.[9]

5.11 References

1. Diu, S. and Gelbier, S. (1987). Dental awareness and attitudes of general medical practitioners. *Community Dental Health*, **4**, 437–444.
2. Seear, J. (1981). *Law and Ethics in Dentistry*. Bristol, Wright, p. 113–114.
3. Central Office of Information. (1990). *A Change in Dental Care for You*. London, HMSO.
4. Yule, B.F., Ryan, M.E. and Parkin, D.W. (1988). Patient charges and the use of dental services: some evidence. *Br. Dent. J.*, Nov., 376–379.
5. *Promoting Better Health: the Government's Programme for Improving Health Care*. (1987). Cm. 249. London, HMSO.
6. *NHS and Community Care Act*. (1990). London, HMSO.
7. Powell, R. (1988). *The Development and Future Direction of the Community Dental Service in England*. Monograph Series. London, University College, University of London.
8. Department of Health and Social Security. (1978). *Health Circular HC(78)14*. London, HMSO.
9. British Dental Association. (1992). *Quality Care for Oral Health*. London, BDA.

Section 2

A Guide to Oral Assessment with Colour Photographs

This section is designed to provide guidance for health care professionals and carers involved in assisting and providing oral care for people, who need some help in meeting their daily oral needs.

For effective goal setting and individualised care, a clear logical approach is required. For effective oral care to take place, the starting point must be assessment of the individual's needs so that care plans can be formulated.

Although clients themselves can often take part in this assessment process, the health professionals are often called upon to use their diagnostic skills. This section is illustrated to show many of the common oral conditions. It is inevitable that photographs cannot always highlight minor changes of colour and texture in membranes. The ability to detect early changes will only develop through experience gained in regular oral examinations. It is recommended that the oral cavity should be examined routinely, so that all health care professionals become acquainted with the healthy mouth in various age groups. The authors have often noticed that nurses dislike examining mouths and giving oral care, in comparison to providing care for other parts of the body! Perhaps a period of intense desensitisation will assist with this barrier.

A number of oral assessment systems are presented so that the most appropriate can be selected. Further research is needed in this area to test and validate criteria.

Improving the standard of oral care requires a systematic approach encompassing training and resources. This section includes an action plan for a key person – the nurse manager – to make this happen. Such a strategy is only likely to succeed with an inter-disciplinary team approach.

Many oral problems are compounded by medications given for other systemic conditions. An overview of the commonest side-effects is given but it should be remembered that this will require constant updating.

The tools for oral care are extensively discussed in this section, so that the most effective can be chosen. Nursing research has identified the deficiencies in many 'oral toilet' procedures, and practical guidance is offered from a dental perspective. For virtually all oral care, the preferred materials are those that the individual would normally use for self-care. Exceptions to this general principle are detailed in Section 3.

6 Oral Assessment

6.1 Introduction
6.2 Types of oral needs
6.3 Key indicators requiring assessment
6.4 Current reported oral assessment systems
6.5 Assessment based on observed and reported behaviour
6.6 Assessment involving the client's views
6.7 Using the outcomes of the oral assessments
6.8 The self-caring individual
6.9 The dependent individual
6.10 Summary
6.11 References

6.1 Introduction

This chapter aims to provide the health professional with assessment tools, so that he or she can define oral needs and identify the standards and objectives for oral care and formulate care plans. Three broad groups of assessment systems are described:

- Those based on health care professionals, usually nurses, using diagnostic skills to assess changes in the oral cavity.
- Assessments that are more behavioural, based on observing clients' activities.
- Assessments that involve the clients' perceptions of their needs.

Oral assessment is required at key stages during any intervention. It is necessary to identify existing oral needs when the patient or client is first seen at the beginning of a period of care. The need for oral care in a dependent person also requires monitoring during the acute phase of illness and later during recovery and rehabilitation.

No single system of oral assessment meets all the criteria currently available; indeed, considering the diversity of oral needs of different client groups, it is unlikely that one system could meet all requirements. A review of those reported in the literature is provided. An assessment system for people in hospital is being piloted and is offered for use by readers of this guide. Most assessment systems will probably require tailoring to specific locations if they are to be sensitive to specific client groups.

The colour plates will help health professionals to assess oral conditions and to make comparisons between healthy and unhealthy mouths.

The illustrations should help alert the health professional to the need for referral to the dental team.

6.2 Types of oral needs

Orodental needs can be classified into three commonly used descriptions of health needs[1]:

- Normative need.
- Felt need.
- Expressed need.

Normative needs (defined by the professional) are ranked very much higher than felt and expressed needs (those needs defined by the client). This has led to a difference in fulfiling these needs, with only the tip of a 'clinical iceberg'[2] having their need met by the health services.

Unmet needs have been shown for all age groups in epidemiological surveys; for example, the level of untreated dental caries in children's teeth and also in the relative minority of people, 43% in the UK, who regularly visit a dentist.[3] There is an even wider gap between normative and expressed needs in the older population.[4,5] As described in Section 1, there are complex reasons why people do not use the dental services, including cultural norms and the presence of barriers such as anxiety and cost.

The important point for health professionals to remember is that they will encounter unmet oral and dental needs in someone presenting with other conditions. These needs will impinge on and affect the general health status and should be addressed.

6.3 Key indicators requiring assessment

The key areas that will give an indication of oral health status and point towards objectives for care include:

- The presence of existing symptoms and signs of orodental disease, including early changes to dental and soft tissues.
- Current mouth care practices and preventive behaviour, including the pattern of dental service attendance.
- The presence of risk factors including systemic disease, medication and disability (see Section 3).
- The presence of key stressors for oral health.

These key areas provide an assessment tool which weighs the different factors, quantifies risk status, and subsequently translates into the degree and type of intervention required.

6.4 Current reported oral assessment systems

Most oral assessment systems seem to have been developed to monitor changes in oral tissues in response to systemic disease or to evaluate nursing interventions. They are mostly diagnostic in approach. Examples include an indicator for stomatitis in acute renal failure[6], patients undergoing chemotherapy[7,8,9], patients in ICU[10], and particularly, elderly dependent people.[11,12] The assessment guides are designed mostly to help nurses carry out mouth care. To monitor the effect of mouth care, Longman and Dewalt[11] developed a guide comprising nine areas (*Table 6.1*).

6.5 Assessment based on observed and reported behaviour

While most hospital-based systems are designed for the nurse or health professional to make an assessment using their clinical expertise, there is also a place for the behavioural approach. If the client's behaviour is measured against a set of objectives over a period of time, a more reliable indicator of dependence can be determined.

This type of system is more appropriate during rehabilitation in a long-stay setting when long-term care and coping strategies are being developed. At this stage, wider involvement of other members of the health care team and carers requires an assessment system that is not purely based on clinical expertise. As assessment of the oral profile has been designed to be incorporated into the Simon Nursing Assessment for the elderly mentally infirm.[17]

The appearance and condition of natural teeth or dentures was also assessed. Each variable was scored between one and three. Longman and Dewalt[11] reported that the system had been tested for reliability and have adapted the system for use by nursing assistants in the USA.

Jenkins[10] used the same variables for patients in ICU and incorporated a number of 'risk factors' which could also be scored to provide an indicator of need (*Table 6.2*).

The effects of chemotherapy on oral health status are problematic[7,9,14], particularly for children.[15] The need for accurate baseline information to allow rapid changes to be measured has been stressed. A highly reliable assessment system (*Table 6.3*), which includes the voice and swallow function, is described by Eilers *et al.*[8]

Whichever assessment system is used, initial training must be given. The amount of time needed to carry out an assessment will vary, for example, the detailed system described by Schweigner takes about 10 minutes[16], while the Dewalt system is much quicker.[13]

Table 6.1 Oral assessment guide for nursing assistants.[11]

A. Amount of salivation	F. Appearance of membranes		
1. Dry	*Tonsillar fossa*	*Cheeks*	*Uvula*
2. Moist	1. Dry	1. Dry	1. Dry
	2. Moist	2. Moist	2. Moist
B. Appearance of tongue	3. Red	3. Red	3. Red
1. Dry	4. Pink	4. Pink	4. Pink
2. Moist	5. Other	5. Other	5. Other
3. Red	(*describe*)		
4. Pink			
5. Other (*describe*)	G. Appearance of lips		
	1. Dry		
C. Appearance of undertongue	2. Moist		
1. Dry	3. Cracked		
2. Moist	4. Rough		
3. Red	5. Smooth		
4. Pink	6. Other (*describe*)		
5. Other (*describe*)			
	H. Appearance of teeth		
D. Appearance of palate	1. Are there natural teeth present? (*If no, proceed to* **I**)		
1. Dry	2. Are any of the teeth:		
2. Moist	a. Intact		
3. Red	b. Broken or cracked		
4. Pink	c. Loose		
5. Other (*describe*)	d. White		
	e. Stained		
E. Appearance of gingival tissues	f. Coated		
1. Dry			
2. Moist	I. Are there dentures present?		
3. Red	a. Full uppers		
4. Pink	b. Full lowers		
5. Other (*describe*)	c. Partial uppers		
	d. Partial lowers		
	e. Cracked or broken		
	f. Smooth		
	g. Rough		

Source: Longman and Dewalt.[11] Reproduced by permission Mosby–Year Book Inc., USA.

Since many factors may affect directly or indirectly a person's ability to maintain oral health, other indicators must be included to assess the level of intervention required. A pilot system (*Figure 6.1*), that identifies non-oral risk factors, has a similar approach to risk calculators for pressure sores. Details of oral abnormalities may be recorded on the oral chart (*Figure 6.2*).

6.6 Assessment involving the client's views

The assessment of orodental needs involving clients themselves has an important role in obtaining a more accurate appreciation of felt and expressed needs. Although undoubtedly there is a gap between the provision of normative need (as assessed by the dental profession) and perceived need (as articulated by the client), it is difficult to say how much of this gap is caused by the inappropriate assessment of normative needs.

Table 6.2 Oral care in the ICU: patient 'at risk'.

Score: 15 and above = two hourly care, 12–14 = hourly care, below 12 = hourly care									
A Patient's age	score	B Normal oral condition	score	C Mastication ability	score	D Nutritional state	score	E Airway	score
16–29	4	Good	4	Full	4	Good	4	Normal	4
30–49	3	Fair	3	Slightly limited	3	Fair	3	Humidified ozygen	3
50–69	2	Poor	2	Very limited	2	Poor	2	ET tube	2
70+	1	Very poor	1	Immobile	1	Very poor	1	Open-mouth breathing	1

If the patient has either/or: (1) Large-dose antibiotics/steroid therapy, (2) Diabetes mellitus, (3) Low HB, (4) Immunosuppression, then the score of 1 should be subtracted from the previous 'at risk' calculator score.

Source: Jenkins.[10] By permission of *Nursing Standard*.

Table 6.3 Oral assessment guide.

Category	Tools for assessment	Methods of measurement	Numerical and descriptive ratings		
			1	2	3
Voice	Auditory	Converse with patient	Normal	Deeper or raspy	Difficult talking or painful
Swallow	Observation	Ask patient to swallow. To test gag reflex, gently place blade on back of tongue and depress	Normal swallow	Some pain on swallow	Unable to swallow
Lips	Visual/palpatory	Observe & feel tissue	Smooth and pink and moist	Dry or cracked	Ulcerated or bleeding
Tongue	Visual/palpatory	Feel and observe appearance of tissue	Pink and moist and papillae present	Coated or loss of papillae with a shiny appearance with or without redness	Blistered or cracked
Saliva	Tongue blade	Insert blade into mouth touching the centre of the tongue and the floor of the mouth	Watery	Thick or raspy	Absent
Mucous membranes	Visual	Observe appearance of tissue	Pink and moist	Reddened or coated (increased whiteness) without ulcerations	Ulcerations with or without bleeding
Gingiva	Tongue blade and visual	Gently press tissue with tip of blade	Pink and stippled and firm	Oedematous with or without redness	Spontaneous bleeding or bleeding with pressure
Teeth or dentures	Visual	Observe appearance of teeth or denture bearing area	Clean and no debris	Plaque or debris in localised areas (between teeth if present)	Plaque or debris generalised along gum line or denture-bearing area

Source: Eilers.[8] Reprinted with permission from the University of Nebraska Medical Center, USA

Name _____   Ward _____

Physical state		Mobility		Dexterity		Mental state		Nutrition/hydration		Oral assessment	N	A
Elective	0	Ambulant	0	Full manual control	0	Alert	0	Normal	0	Lips	0	1
Convalescence	1	Walks with aid	1	Slightly limited	1	Apathetic/overactive	1	Soft/liquid diet	1	Tongue	0	1
Rehabilitation	2	Walks with help	2	Poor co-ordination	2	Confused/psychotic	2	Nil by mouth/limited oral fluids, e.g. hourly	2	Mucous membranes	0	1
Acute illness	3	Chair bound	3	Very limited	3	Stuporous	3	Dehydrated/nausea/vomiting	3	Saliva	0	1
Chronic illness/chronic cancer	4	Bedfast	4	Paralysis/absent limb	4			Refusal of intake	4	Gingiva	0	1
										Teeth	0	1
										Dentures	0	1

High risk

				Score	
02 Therapy/dyspnoeic patients	5	Spinal injury	10	18–38	Dependent
Unconscious/intubated	5	Chronic mental illness	5	11–17	Assistance
Mild mental handicap	5	Acute mental illness	10	6–10	Prompting/minimal assistance
Severe mental handicap	10	Age under 6 years	5	0– 5	Self care
Diabetes	5	Age 70+	5		
Radiotherapy	5	Terminal care	10		
Radiotherapy head and neck	10	CVAs	5		
Chemotherapy	10	Physical handicap	5		
Immune compromised/MND	5				

Total score............   Date............   Signature (primary nurse)............

Figure 6.1 Pilot scheme for oral assessment.

Holistic Oral Care

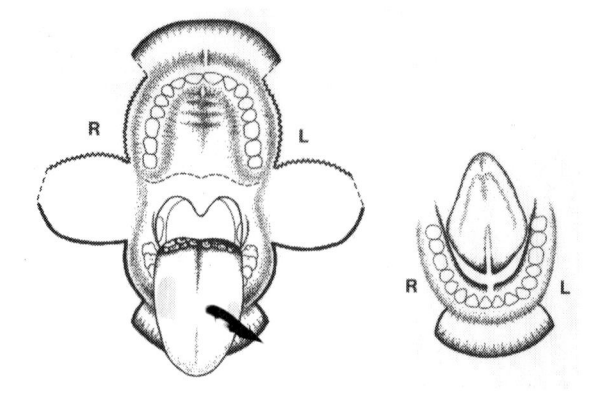

Figure 6.2 Oral chart.

Hoad-Reddick[18] reviewed the differences between perceived need and normative need in a wide cross-section of studies; the differences ranged between 12–49%. It is axiomatic that any measurement of need which includes the views of the client is likely to be more sensitive. In Hoad-Reddick's study, the need for treatment as assessed by a list of four questions (*Table 6.4*) and a simple visual examination by care workers was found to correlate closely with the need for treatment as assessed by a dental professional.[18]

Table 6.4 Client's assessment of oral needs.[18]

1. Do you think you need any dental treatment?
   Type of treatment needed:
   Restorative/denture adjustment/denture replacement
2. Do you have any painful areas in your mouth?
3. Do you have any problems eating?
4. When did you last visit a dentist?
   Or how old are your dentures?
   No idea   < 2yrs   3–5 yrs
   6–10 yrs   > 10 yrs

Source: Hoade-Reddick.[18] *By permission of Munskgard International Publishers Ltd., Copenhagen, Denmark.*

6.7 Using the outcomes of oral assessments

Whichever assessment is used, a primary objective is to indicate how much assistance an individual requires to maintain oral health at a particular time. The health care professional is likely to encounter large numbers of people needing varying amounts of assistance.

6.8 The self-caring individual

In the case of individuals in a hospital or institution, their very presence indicates a state of dependence, however temporary. If they are self-caring with respect to their oral health, the role of the health care professional is to ensure that they have access to the necessary equipment and facilities summarised in *Table 6.5*.

The procedures that the individual should be encouraged to follow are described in Chapter 2 for adults, and Chapter 3 for children.

6.9 The dependent individual

The degree of dependence will vary from individual to individual and in response to the patient's systemic condition. However, when oral care has to be undertaken by a health care professional, i.e. the patient is totally dependent for oral needs, the following procedure is suggested (*Table 6.6*). It is based on a system currently in use.[19] Gloves should be worn for all procedures involving contact with oral tissues and for handling dentures.

Table 6.5 Equipment and facilities needed by the self-caring adult for oral care.

Mouth and tooth-cleaning equipment:
- Toothbrush
- Toothpaste
- Dental floss or other interdental cleaners if used
- Denture-cleaning brush
- Denture cleaner

Access to suitable facilities:
- Suitable privacy
- Clean running water
- Mirror at appropriate position
- Glass or receptacle for rinsing
- Container for dentures and other appliances or prostheses

Access to suitable information and advice:
- Information regarding facilities
- Services available
- Appropriate preventive advice

Holistic Oral Care

Table 6.6 Oral care procedures in the dependent individual.

Oral care for the dentate (natural teeth)

1. Toothbrushing.
   - Teeth and gums should be brushed.
   - Use a small soft toothbrush and a pea-sized amount of fluoride toothpaste.
   - Clean all surfaces to remove plaque and food debris, paying particular attention to buccal and lingual surfaces.
   - Any excess may be removed by rinsing, if this is permitted, or swabbing with a gloved finger wrapped in gauze.
   - Chlorhexidine gluconate dental gel (1%) may be prescribed and used in the same way as toothpaste.
2. Towelling.
   - If the patient is at risk from toothbrushing, i.e. dysphagic, the teeth and gums should be swabbed using a gloved finger wrapped in gauze soaked in chlorhexidine gluconate dental gel (1%) or chlorhexidine gluconate mouthwash (0.2%).
   - Gentle friction is very effective at removing food debris when toothbrushing is difficult.
3. Mouthwashing.
   If access to the patient's mouth is difficult, but the patient is able to rinse safely, the nurse should assist the patient by:
   - Dispensing chlorhexidine gluconate mouthwash.
   - Assisting the patient whilst rinsing.
   - Supplying a receptacle to receive used mouthwash. A straw or adapted beaker may be helpful.

Oral care of mucosa, lips and tongue (dentate and edentulous)

1. Remove any dentures.
2. Mucosa and tongue may be cleaned by gentle brushing with a small soft toothbrush.
3. Where cleaning is not possible, the mucosa and tongue may be cleaned by swabbing with a gloved finger wrapped in gauze soaked in chlorhexidine gluconate mouthwash (0.2%).
4. If the patient is capable of rinsing safely, then the nurse should help the patient rinse with chlorhexidine gluconate mouthwash (0.2%).
5. In patients who have little saliva (xerostomia), or whose saliva is of abnormal consistency, either thin and watery or thick and viscous:
   - Small sips of iced water.
   - Small sips of saliva substitute.
   - The mouth should be swabbed with a saliva substitute.
   - Atomised water sprays may be helpful.
6. Lips may be bathed with saline and lubricated with a lanolin-based cream.

Care of dentures

1. Denture cleaning.
   - Remove dentures twice daily and brush thoroughly with a toothbrush or denture brush and unperfumed soap or chlorhexidine gluconate cleansing solution.
   - Clean dentures over a basin of cold water to prevent them breaking if they are dropped.
   - Rinse thoroughly in cold water and return dentures to the mouth.
2. Hard deposits or stains not removed by brushing may require professional cleaning. Contact the dental team.
3. Remove dentures at night and, after cleaning, place in a receptacle of cold water.
4. Plastic dentures should not be soaked overnight in effervescent cleansers. Chlorhexidine mouthwash may be used to soak dentures when disinfection is necessary, but the dentures will become stained. Chlorine-based cleaners corrode metal dentures and may bleach plastic dentures if used constantly.
5. Dentures must be kept moist when not being worn.
6. If the patient insists on wearing dentures at night, ensure that the mouth and dentures are scrupulously clean, and that the patient knows that continuous wear is harmful to the mouth.
7. Partial dentures need extra attention in cleaning to ensure that food and plaque are removed efficiently. Teeth in contact with the denture and denture clasps are more prone to decay, unless both teeth and denture are kept clean and free from plaque.
8. Patients should be strongly discouraged from wearing a partial denture at night.
9. Dentures with a soft lining should be brushed very gently and may be cleaned with a dilute solution of bicarbonate of soda. Denture cleaners should not be used as they may damage the soft lining.

6.10 Summary

Three types of assessment systems are described. The first is assessment of changes in the oral cavity by nurses, and is mainly used for the dependent patient. As well as changes in the mouth, other risk factors for oral health are identified. Examples in the nursing literature are reviewed and a prototype assessment is offered for use.

The second type of assessment is behavioural and based on what clients can do. These systems can be used in a multi-disciplinary context as the outcomes may involve different health professionals working together.

The third type of assessment involves the client's own perception of their orodental needs. A series of oral care procedures for the dependent patient are included.

6.11 References

1. Bradshaw, J. (1972). A taxonomy of social need. In: McLachlan G. (Ed.) *Problems and progress in medical care: essays on current research.* Oxford, Oxford University Press, pp. 69–72.
2. Last, J. (1963). The clinical iceberg: completing the clinical picture in general practice. *Lancet*, ii, 28–31.
3. Todd, J. *et al.* (1982). *Adult Dental Health. Vol 2: UK 1978.* London, HMSO.
4. Smith, J. and Sheiham, A. (1980). Dental treatment needs and demands of an elderly population in England. *Comm. Dent. Oral Epidemiol.*, **8**, 360–364.
5. Hoad-Reddick, G., Grant A.A. and Griffiths, C.S. (1987). Knowledge of dental services provided: investigations in an elderly population. *Comm. Dent. Oral Epidemiol.*, **15**, 137–140.
6. Ginsberg, M.K. (1961). A study of oral hygiene nursing care. *Am. J. Nursing*, **61**, 67–69.
7. Richardson, A. (1987). A process standard for oral care. *Nursing Times*, Aug. 12, **83**(32), 38–40.
8. Eilers, J., Berger, A.M. and Peterson, M.C. (1988). Development, testing and application of the oral assessment guide. *Oncology Nursing Forum*, **15**(3), 325–330.
9. Crosby, C. (1989). Method in mouth care. *Nursing Times*, Aug. 30, **35**, 38–41.
10. Jenkins, D. (1989). Oral care in the ICU: an important nursing role. *Nursing Standard*, **4**(7), 24–28.
11. Longman, A.J. and Dewalt, E.M. (1986). A guide of oral assessment. *Geriatric Nursing*, Sept./Oct., 252–253.
12. Blaney, G.M. (1986). Mouth care – basic and essential. *Geriatric Nursing*, Sept./Oct., 242–243.
13. DeWalt, E. (1975). Effects of timed hygiene measures on oral mucosa in a group of elderly subjects. *Nr. Research*, **24**, 104–108.
14. Bersani, G. and Carl, W. (1983). Oral care for cancer patients. *Am. J. Nursing*, **4**, 533–536.

15. Campbell, S. (1987). Mouth care in cancer patients. Spotlight on children. *Nursing Times*, **83**(29), 59–60.
16. Schweiger, J.L. *et al.* (1980). Oral assessment: how to do it. *Am. J. Nursing*, **80**, 654–657.
17. O'Donovan, S. (1992). Simon's nursing assessment. *Nursing Times*, **88**(2) 30–33.
18. Hoad-Reddick, G. (1991). A study to determine oral health needs of institutionalised elderly patients by non-dental health care workers. *Comm. Dent. Oral Epidemiol.*, **19**, 233–236.
19. South Glamorgan Health Authority. (1990). *Unit 3 Policy on Percutaneous Endoscopic Gastrostomy. Appendix 1*. Cardiff, SGHA.

7 Role of the Nurse Manager in Promoting Oral Care

7.1 Introduction
7.2 Development of an oral health strategy
7.3 Continuing education and training for the nursing team
7.4 A ward or community-based programme: a case for oral care
7.5 The interdisciplinary approach
7.6 Keeping the issue of oral care on the agenda
7.7 Putting the strategy into action: providing the training
7.8 Meeting the training needs of the whole team
7.9 What to include in the training programme
7.10 The requirements at ward or community level for self-care
7.11 The requirements when assistance is needed
7.12 Summary
7.13 References

7.1 Introduction

The role of the nurse manager, either at ward or community level, is pivotal in making things happen. It is essential that the whole issue of oral care is addressed at this level to ensure that the different activities and professions are brought together to maintain a good standard of oral care at the interface with the patient or client. It is the nursing team, led by its manager, which has the intimate knowledge of individual patients' needs, and which is responsible for the patients' continuing, rather than episodic, care.

Good oral care is more than ensuring adequate access to dental professionals for treatment, even though this baseline level of service is difficult enough to obtain in many areas of health care. Although oral health care may not be the primary reason for the patient's initial referral for nursing care, unmet oral needs are found in many groups of patients. These needs may not have been expressed, and a nursing strategy is required to examine oral health needs and to provide the mechanisms to meet them. This applies not just to the period of nursing care, but also to helping patients develop coping strategies to maintain their oral health. This chapter sets out the areas of an effective oral health strategy, and then discusses the practical contents of such programmes.

7.2 Development of an oral health strategy

An effective oral health strategy will contain several key elements. These include the use of effective oral assessment criteria at the start of care because many patient groups – the elderly being a very good example[1] – have low expressed oral needs. Chapter 6 has described some of the current criteria used. However, it is important that these criteria are linked to clear nursing objectives.

7.3 Continuing education and training for the nursing team

Oral care has a low status in the present training of nurses, and so it is important to address the issue of continuing education programmes for all staff grades. As nursing care is increasingly provided by a team approach, it is vital that training and education are provided to all team members, particularly the non-professionally trained who are more likely to be involved with meeting the daily needs of highly dependent patients.

Training for these groups is particularly important because, as with any task-oriented group, their original training may have lacked the conceptual understanding of the need for oral care. Even though the professionally trained nurse may have done the oral assessment for a patient and set care goals, the non-professional team members may not have the skills to implement the tasks set. This may seem obvious to the point of farce, but it is easy to overlook the fact that our personal oral care skills are not always appropriate for those in our care, and that specialist approaches may be needed.

The importance of continuing education to provide a regular update of oral needs is becoming increasingly apparent both within the dental profession and in the wider health professions. Changes in oral health status, as described in Chapter 1, will mean that client groups will have different oral health needs to those of their stereotypical portrayal. For example, increasing numbers of older people are retaining their teeth into later life in most industrialised countries.[2]

Specific risk groups for dental and oral disease are emerging. Most available research data on oral care carried out by nurses have been on

Role of the Nurse Manager

patients with cancer or those in intensive care units. This may be because in these specific areas, oral care is more problematic and deficiencies in oral care produce overt problems, e.g. mucositis. For many client groups in nursing care, whether continuing or short-term, oral care is a quality-of-life issue (see Section 3 on oral handicap and disability).

Methods of providing oral care, the most appropriate tools, and the degree of oral care required, are issues that need to be addressed.[3,4] Nursing research has pointed out the inadequate scientific basis of many existing procedures.[5]

One of the primary aims of this guide is to provide a core of knowledge for use in continuing education and training; the first section provided the basic knowledge and skills needed, while Section 3 highlights the particular needs of different client groups.

7.4 A ward or community-based programme: a case for oral care

Implementation of hospital-based or district-based policies and guidelines at field level is a task clearly within the remit of the nurse manager. It is fair to state that there are few areas of nursing care in which there are not many competing pressures for nursing time and resources. This is a situation unlikely to change in the future, as demographic changes in most industrialised societies tend towards an ageing population presenting greater demands. However, effective oral care need not be time-consuming. Certainly, where it is practised in a 'hands-on' manner, it can be made more effective without increasing the time needed. The nurse manager is in the position of being able to balance the needs of the client group with the individual's needs and with the rationing of staff and non-staff resources. The likely outcomes of an effective oral assessment will be in three main areas (*Table 7.1*).

Table 7.1 Oral assessment: areas of need.

- A health promotion need for the nurse to help the individual develop more effective oral self-care skills.
- A treatment need requiring the intervention of the dental professional.
- A need for assistance with oral care in the short or long term for the individual with a degree of dependence to meet their daily needs.

7.5 The interdisciplinary approach

The compartmentalised approach to the delivery of health care in most countries means that many members of the health care team work in isolation of each other, and that interdisciplinary co-operation exists in theory rather than practice. The primary health care approach[6] has been

Holistic Oral Care

one solution, but in any organisation there are a number of key people employed to bring others together. The nurse manager is placed in a position to control the whole process (*Figure 7.1*).

Nurse provides: The assessment of needs Formation of goals	←	Nurse manager provides: Access to training Nurse time

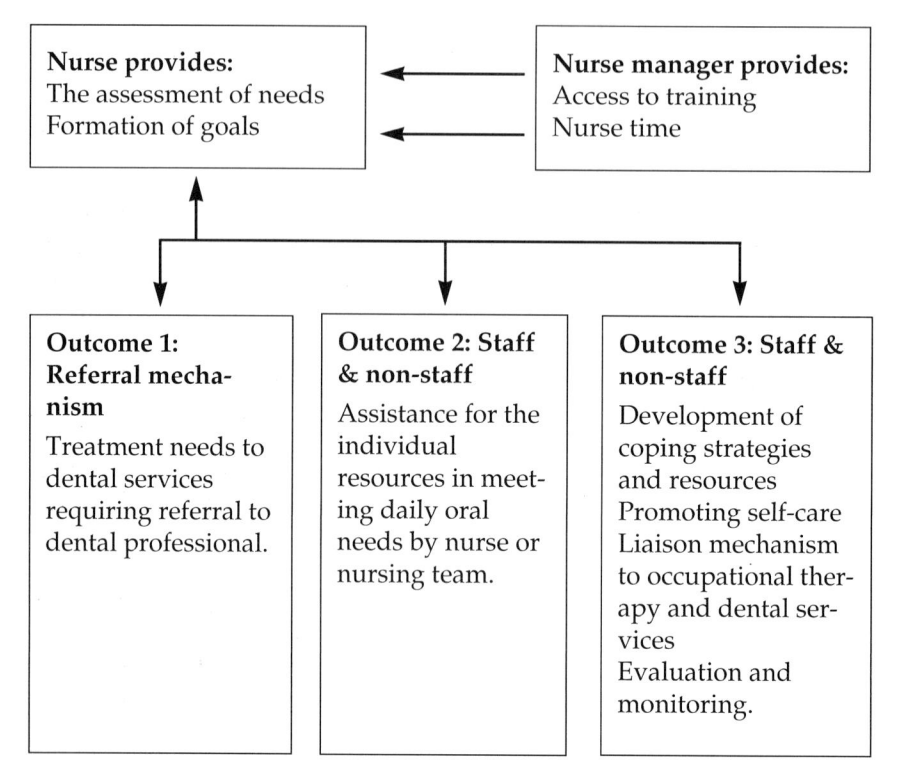

Outcome 1: Referral mechanism Treatment needs to dental services requiring referral to dental professional.	Outcome 2: Staff & non-staff Assistance for the individual resources in meeting daily oral needs by nurse or nursing team.	Outcome 3: Staff & non-staff Development of coping strategies and resources Promoting self-care Liaison mechanism to occupational therapy and dental services Evaluation and monitoring.

Figure 7.1 The individual with oral needs.

7.6 Keeping the issue of oral care on the agenda

The evaluation and revisiting of individual objectives in care plans will note the changes in the status of the patient as he or she moves through the process of treatment to rehabilitation to recovery.

This will be accompanied by changes in oral status and oral needs as drug therapy changes and the individual becomes more self-reliant or develops coping skills. An efficient referral mechanism is required as the changes in oral status may necessitate interventions by the dental team.

7.7 Putting the strategy into action: providing the training

Whichever oral assessment procedure is selected as most appropriate, it is likely that there will be a training need to ensure required staff are conversant with its use. Sufficient research into current nurse-based oral- and mouth-care practices has been done to show that many existing procedures are outdated, ineffective and based on non-empirical findings.[3,4,5]

The reason for many of these shortcomings lies in poor communication within the dental profession, which has failed to involve itself sufficiently in the formulation and review of procedures. Despite a challenge to the dental profession to be involved in training from several seminal nurse-based research articles[3,4], there have been only a few reported programmes in which there has been close co-operation between the nursing and dental professions in training and devising programmes.

O'Laughlin[7] describes a programme for a residential home for the elderly which included training for nursing staff involving their own personal oral skills. A similar approach was used in the primary training of nurses in a programme taught by community dental staff.[8] The rationale behind this approach was that improvement of personal oral practices would lead to greater competency in the oral care of clients. But, since the practice of effective oral care requires modification of care to the client's needs, it is questionable whether this approach is appropriate as it may not encourage objectivity in assessment. However, it does provide an excellent starting point, and if appropriately handled can help to minimise some of the barriers and negative views that mouth care seems to produce among nurses.

7.8 Meeting the training needs of the whole team

When training needs are being reviewed, the needs of those working shifts and nights should be considered and programmes should be timetabled to include these.[9]

The specialist content for the training can be obtained from the dental team, but the nurse manager should specify training needs very clearly so that the programme is orientated to the client group being cared for. It will be a more efficient use of training resources if nurse trainers themselves undergo this oral training so that the knowledge and skills received can be 'cascaded' throughout the team. As with all practical skills, adequate provision for hands-on training is essential, and in the learning environment the group itself can provide this opportunity by practising on each other's mouths. The dental hygienist is the key member of the dental team with regard to the practical aspects of mouth care.

7.9 What to include in the training programme

Content of the training programme should be tailored to meet the oral health issues of the specific client group. However, there will be a common core component. We suggest that the core knowledge as found in Chapter 2 is an essential starting point, followed by the sections for the relevant client group. It is worth noting that most adults will already feel they have a reasonable level of competency in personal oral practices and will need opportunities for practice and consideration before adapting. A small group approach, which allows students to explore their own dental views, and their anxieties, will be more successful. For example, many health care professionals have an aversion to handling dentures.[10]

It is also suggested that the oral needs of the client group be covered in a separate session to highlight the modifications and special approaches that may be needed.

7.10 The requirements at ward or community level for self-care

The requirements at ward or community level will be moderated by the needs of the client group and the degree of oral self-care found. Except for the very few patients who are totally dependent, patients will themselves be involved in the care of their own mouths.

There are a number of central requirements which the nurse manager can ensure are met in order to minimise barriers to oral care. These include the physical requirements:

- Access to clean, preferably running, water and to a sink.
- Access to a suitable mirror and adequate illumination.
- Access to appropriate equipment: toothbrushes, denture brushes, cleaning pastes, dental floss, woodsticks, and any modifications to meet special needs.
- Access to dental services for screening and treatment.

Other requirements include flexibility of ward routines so that oral care can follow the individual's own established routines of mouth care. For example, some people prefer to clean their mouths after breakfast, others before. In order to normalise the situation as much as possible, ward routines should not be so rigid as to prevent this.

Even young children are likely to be socialised into a fairly fixed routine as to when, where, and how they practice mouth care, and it can be disorientating to introduce them to a system that changes these patterns. With older established patterns, routines will be even more difficult to change. If the objective is to promote self-care the first step must be the provision of facilities that will allow individuals to re-establish, as much as possible, their previous patterns.

Although orientated to the ward setting, this checklist can easily be applied to the home as part of a community assessment.

7.11 The requirements when assistance is needed

If the oral assessment indicates that some help will be needed with oral care in either the short term or long term, a care plan should be made. As the oral health status will change in response to systemic factors, so the type and degree of self-care will alter. The nurse manager should be satisfied that care plans are appropriate and reviewed.

For example, a client who has had a cerebrovascular accident will pass through several stages of oral dependency. Initially, he or she may be semiconscious and fed intravenously or parentally. At this stage, oral needs will consist of a safe receptacle for dentures, which at this point should be labelled and stored wet in a named container, and the mouth will require oral toilet and frequent moistening for comfort.

As recovery continues and eating is begun, the presence of any hemiplegia means that the patient will need help in cleaning both mouth and dentures. Food is likely to accumulate in the mouth and it may be difficult to retain dentures. The temporary use of fixative can be helpful at this stage until a dentist can make an assessment. Adaptions to denture-cleaning brushes may also be needed, while a dentate client will need help with toothbrushing.

Any residual loss of function may require permanent modification of dentures and of cleaning equipment for dentures or teeth. It is also possible that, due to large unmet oral needs, the nurse will discover other long-standing problems or pathology which merit a referral to the dental team. In the community setting, this may entail nurses themselves facilitating referral and subsequent treatment.

7.12 Summary

In this chapter, the central role of the nurse manager in both the ward and the community setting has been addressed. Although much of the practical work involves others, the nurse, the nurse trainer, the nursing team, the occupational therapist, the dental team, etc., it is the nurse manager who is the lynchpin around whom good nursing practice revolves.

7.13 References

1. Smith, J.M. and Sheiham, A. (1979). How dental conditions handicap the elderly. *Comm. Dent. Oral Epidemiol.*, **7**, 305–310.
2. World Health Organisation. (1985). *Oral Health Care Systems: an international collaborative study*. London, Quintessence.
3. Howarth, H. (1977). Mouth care procedures for the very ill. *Nursing Times*, March 10, **73**, 346–347.
4. Sammon, P., Page, C. and Shepherd, G. (1987). Oral hygiene. *Nursing Times*, May 13, **83**(19), 25–27.
5. Trenter Roth, P. and Creason, N.S. (1986). Nurse-administered oral hygiene: is there a scientific basis? *J. Advanced Nurs.*, **11**, 323–331.
6. World Health Organisation. (1984). *Health Promotion. A discussion document on the concept and principles*. Copenhagen, WHO.
7. O'Laughlin, J.M. (1986). A dental program for nursing home residents. *Geriatr. Nurs.*, (NY)., Sept–Oct., **7**(5), 248–250.
8. Munday, P. and Gelbier, S. (1984). Provision of dental health education in nurse training. *Nurse Education Today*, **3**(6), 124–125.
9. Nelson, J. (1988). Continuing education at night. *Geriatric Nursing and Home Care*, **8**(1), 9–10.
10. Boyle, S.J. (1990). A study of mouth care practices in a long-stay hospital for the elderly. MSc thesis. University of Manchester.

COLOUR PLATES

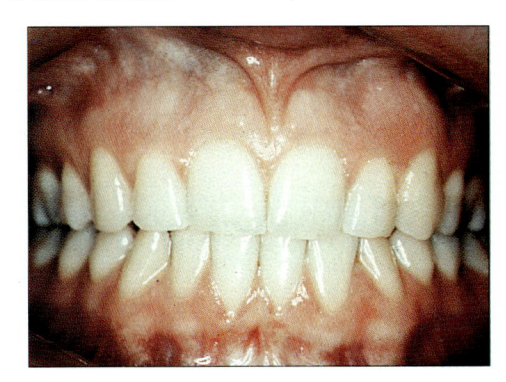

Colour Plate 1. Healthy adult mouth. Gingivae (gums) are pale pink and firm. Teeth are regular and meet normally.

Colour Plate 2. An 88-year-old self-caring male retaining most teeth with some recession of the gingivae and toothbrush abrasion at the gingival margins. The biting surfaces show attrition and there is some evidence of gingivitis. However, this is a relatively healthy mouth. The subject wears a skeleton design metal denture to restore occlusal contact.

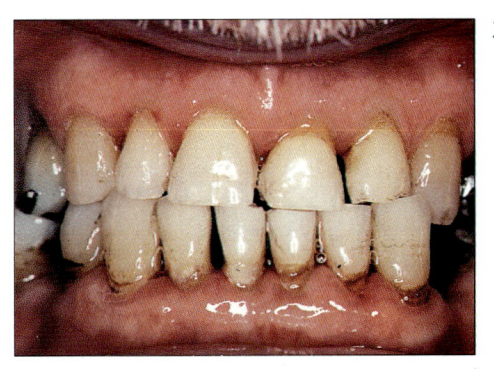

Colour Plate 3. Gingivitis in a young male with learning difficulties. The areas of enamel opacity may have been caused by decayed primary teeth affecting developing secondary teeth or may be related to neonatal illness or trauma.

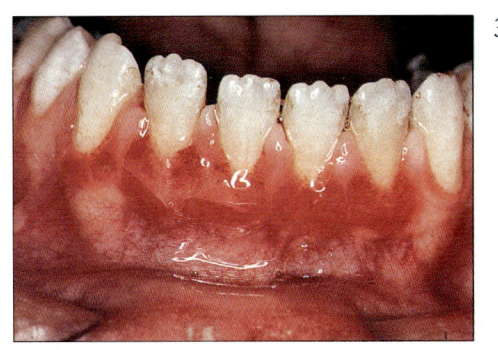

Colour Plate 4. Gingival recession with chronic periodontal disease leading to mobility of the two lower central teeth. Calculus is visible on the roots.

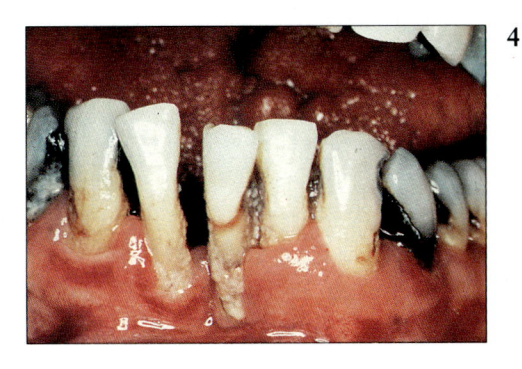

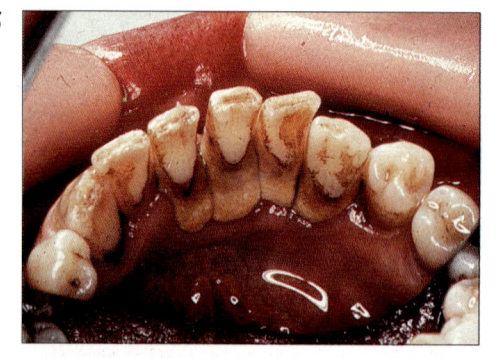

Colour Plate 5. Calculus and staining behind the lower front teeth. This is an area prone to calculus because of its proximity to the sublingual salivary glands.

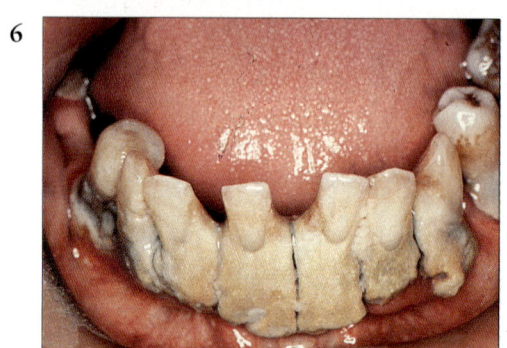

Colour Plate 6. Very heavy deposits of calculus on the lower front teeth, evidence of poor oral hygiene and dental neglect.

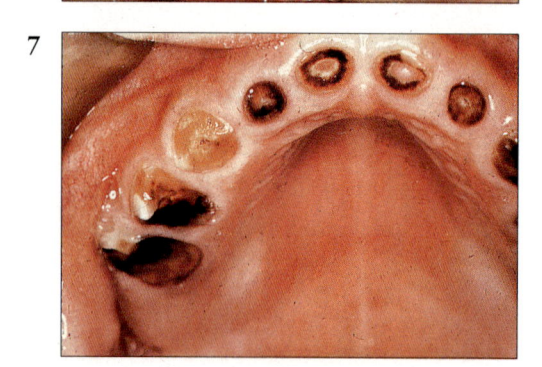

Colour Plate 7. Bottle caries in the upper primary teeth of a three-year-old child.

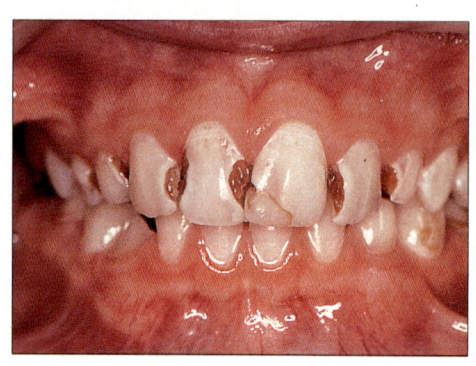

Colour Plate 8. Advanced caries in the mixed dentition of a nine-year-old child. Cavities are easily visible between the four upper front teeth; these are the secondary teeth which have only been present for a few years. The child had a dietary history of at least nine cans of carbonated drinks daily and never drank any other liquids.

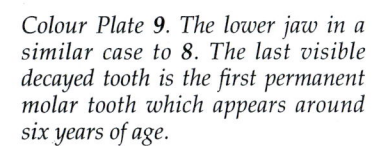

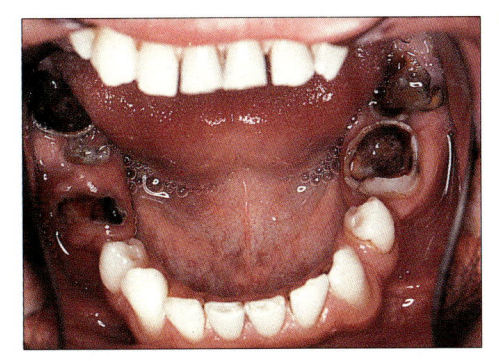

Colour Plate 9. The lower jaw in a similar case to 8. The last visible decayed tooth is the first permanent molar tooth which appears around six years of age.

Colour Plate 10. An elderly male whose oral and dental problems were identified as the result of admission to hospital following a cerebrovascular accident. There are signs of gingival recession, cervical (root) caries and deficient fillings.

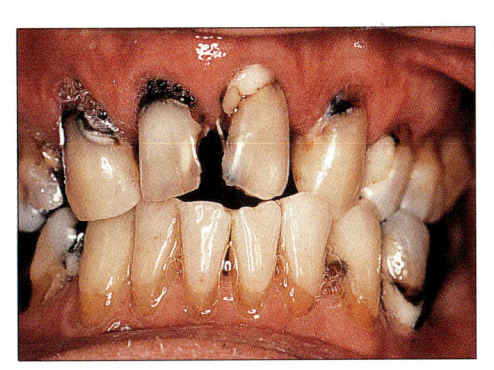

Colour Plate 11. Radiation caries which characteristically encircles the necks of the teeth.

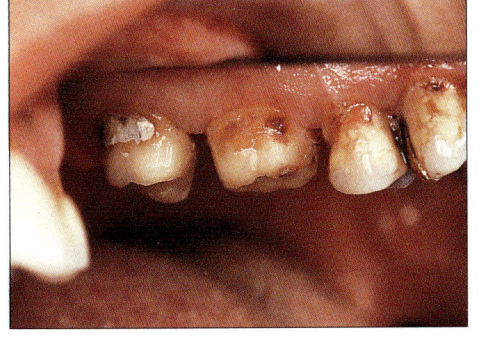

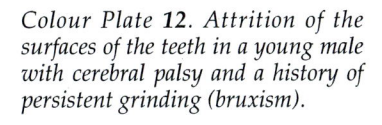

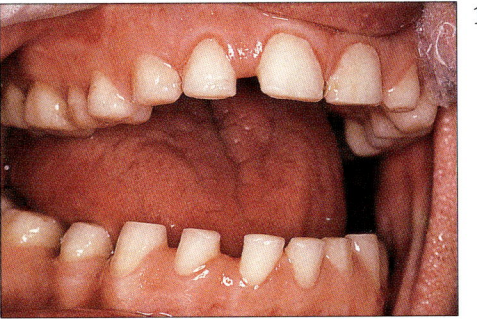

Colour Plate 12. Attrition of the surfaces of the teeth in a young male with cerebral palsy and a history of persistent grinding (bruxism).

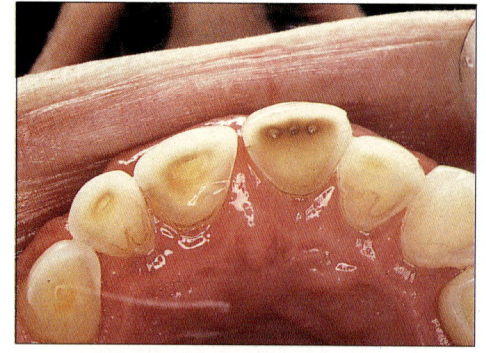

Colour Plate 13. Erosion of the palatal surfaces of teeth caused by persistent acid regurgitation.

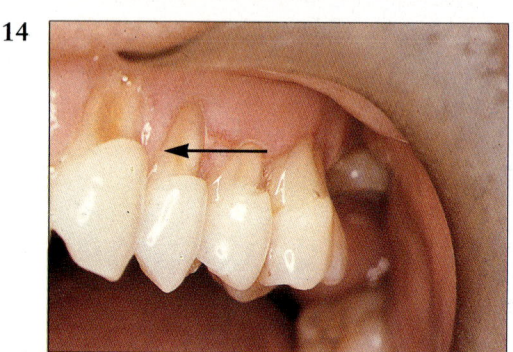

Colour Plate 14. Abrasion caused by excessive horizontal toothbrushing, 'sawing' into the weaker dentine at the gum margin.

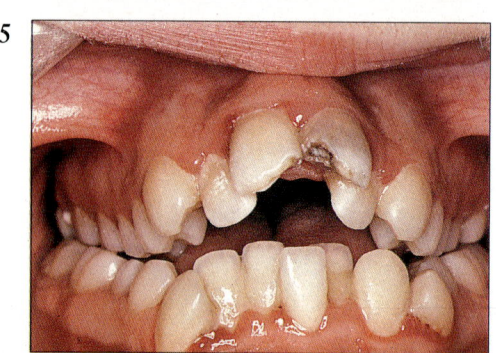

Colour Plate 15. Malocclusion in a 14-year-old female with a learning difficulty. Early intervention to extract teeth would have reduced the degree of overcrowding, although orthodontic treatment would not have been appropriate due to poor compliance and co-operation. A fractured upper central tooth is decayed suggesting lack of dental treatment.

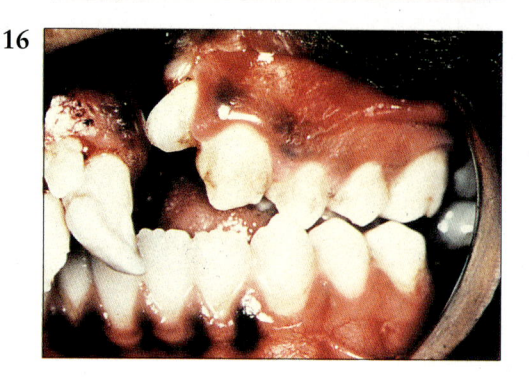

Colour Plate 16. Cleft lip and palate in a young male immigrant who had not been given early surgical treatment in his native land. Facial disfigurement and embarrassment while eating had led to psychological problems and withdrawal. These problems started to resolve after cosmetic surgical repair.

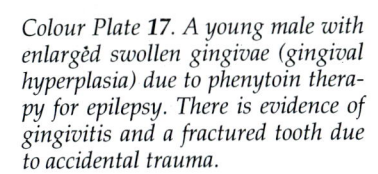

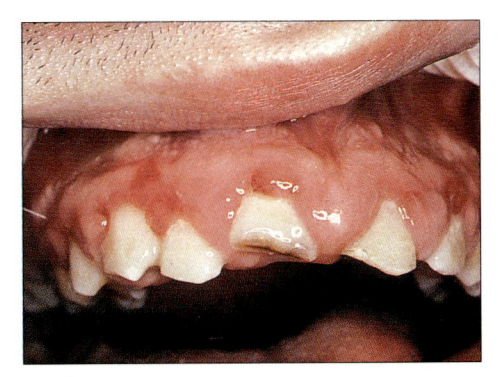

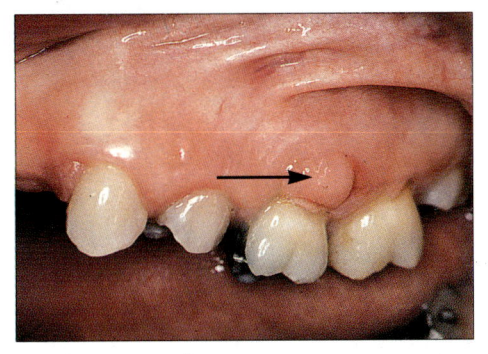

Colour Plate 17. A young male with enlarged swollen gingivae (gingival hyperplasia) due to phenytoin therapy for epilepsy. There is evidence of gingivitis and a fractured tooth due to accidental trauma.

Colour Plate 18. Swelling of the gingivae, a side-effect of nifedipine.

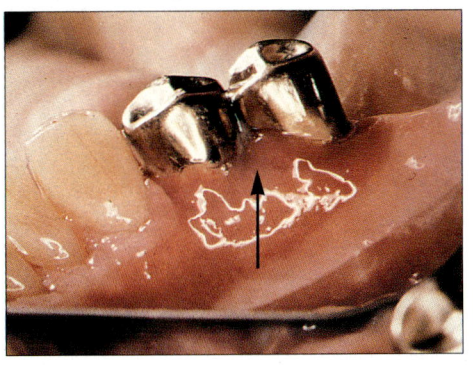

Colour Plate 19. Aspirin burn: a red inflamed area of gingivae next to the crowned teeth caused by placing an aspirin tablet there for local pain relief.

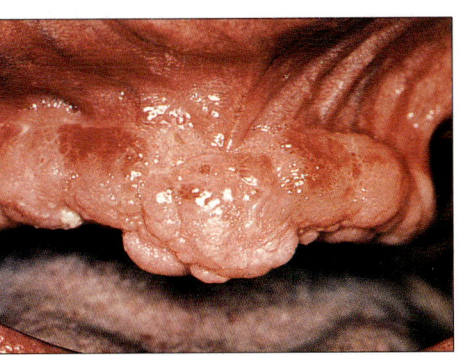

Colour Plate 20. Hyperplasia (swelling and enlargement) and inflammation in a denture wearer taking cyclosporin.

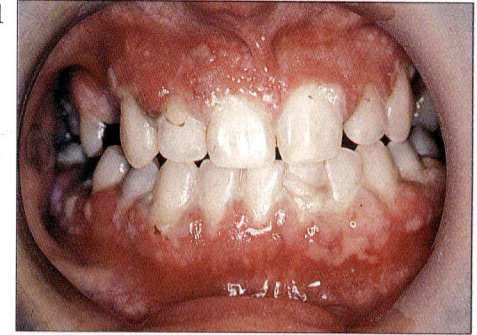

Colour Plate 21. Herpes stomatitis.

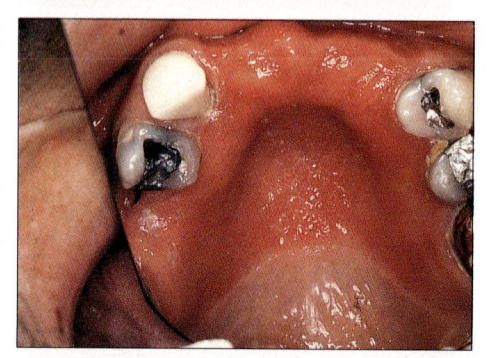

Colour Plate 22. Denture stomatitis: red areas of the palate caused by contact with a partial upper denture. Patients rarely complain of soreness and may be completely unaware of the condition. It is mainly due to candidal infection and is associated with poor denture hygiene and wearing dentures at night.

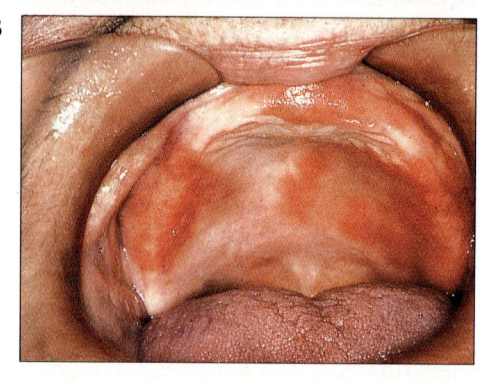

Colour Plate 23. Candidal infection of the palate in a diabetic patient who wore a complete upper denture.

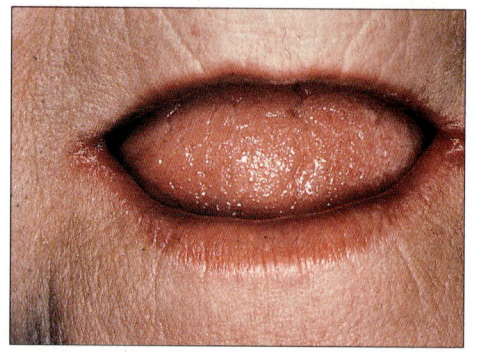

Colour Plate 24. Candidal infection of the commissures (angular cheilitis).

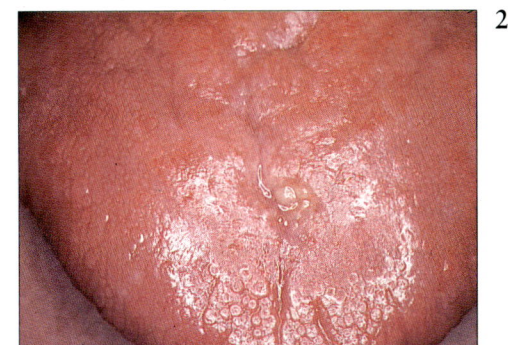

Colour Plate 25. Candidal infection of the tongue.

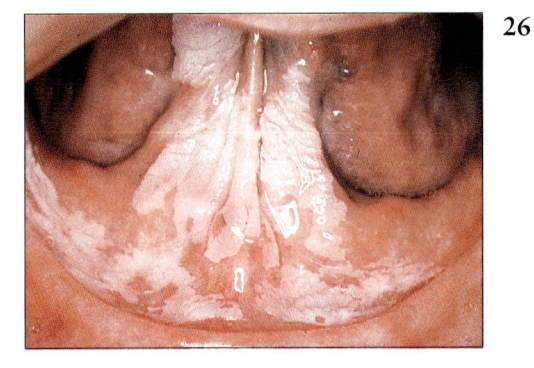

Colour Plate 26. Sublingual keratosis: a dense white keratinised area in the floor of the mouth under the tongue.

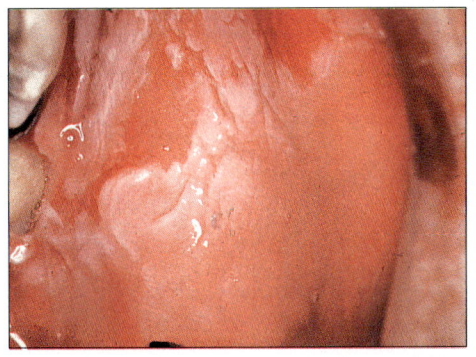

Colour Plate 27. Leukoplakia of the buccal mucosa.

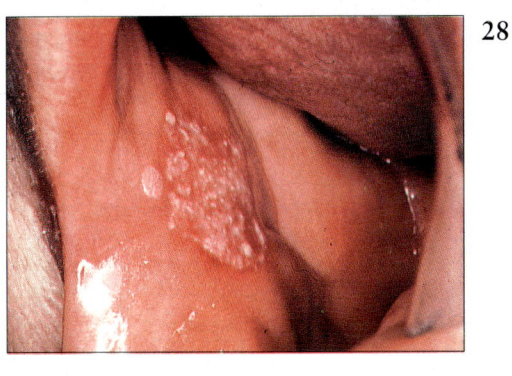

Colour Plate 28. Red and white patches on the buccal mucosa; this relatively innocuous-looking lesion is malignant.

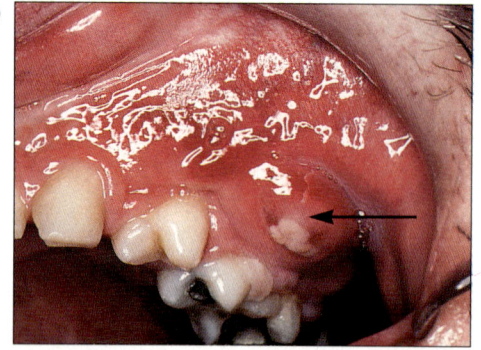

Colour Plate 29. Carcinoma of the maxilla.

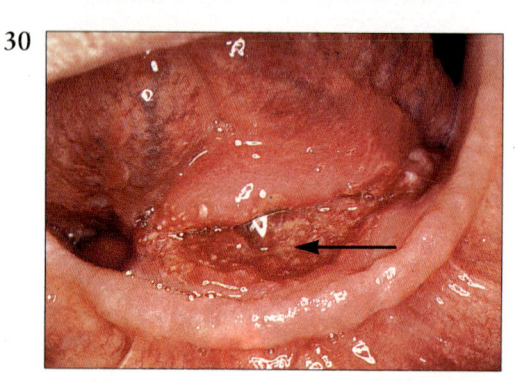

Colour Plate 30. Carcinoma of the floor of the mouth; the patient complained of soreness from rubbing by dentures and an ulcer which would not heal.

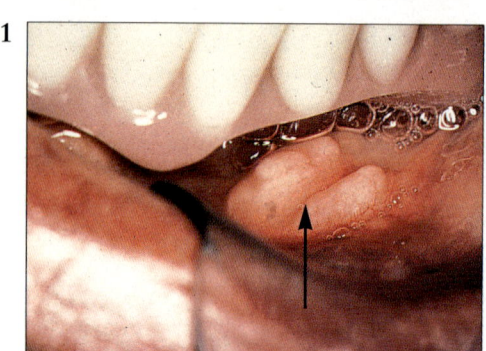

Colour Plate 31. Denture granuloma caused by ill-fitting dentures.

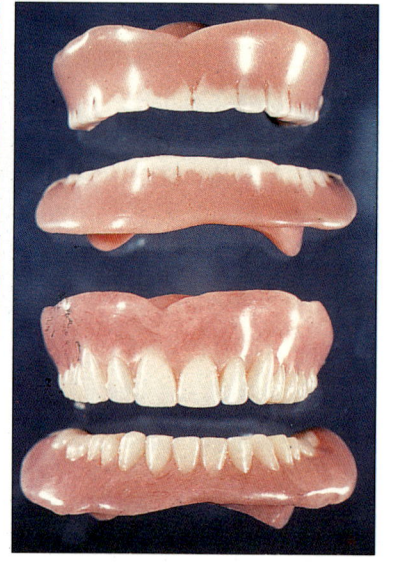

Colour Plate 32. Old and new dentures.

8 Oral Effects of Medication

8.1 Introduction
8.2 Sugar in medicines
8.3 Contact reactions
8.4 Drugs in pregnancy
8.5 Oral side-effects
8.6 Summary
8.7 References

8.1 Introduction

The principles of good pharmacotherapy involve balancing the benefits of medication against the potential risks and side-effects. Age, body weight, liver and kidney disease affect toxicity and the rate at which drugs are excreted from the body. The problem of compliance and the possibility of abuse must be considered. Tissues which exhibit rapid cell growth and cell turnover are more likely to be affected by drug side-effects. Blood cells and the cellular surface tissues of the mouth fall into this category.

The mouth is permanently populated by micro-organisms: bacteria, fungi and viruses. In the healthy individual with good oral hygiene and normal salivary flow, a fairly constant balance is achieved between different micro-organisms with no evidence of oral infection. However, an upset in the balance of micro-organisms caused by illness or medication may lead to oral infection. The importance of saliva and its antibacterial effects is summarised in Chapter 1.

Drugs may also have a direct effect upon oral tissues and more importantly on the developing foetus, if taken in pregnancy. This chapter summarises the more important oral side-effects of medication.

8.2 Sugar in medicines

An area of particular concern to the dental profession is the use of extrinsic sugars to make drug preparations more palatable and acceptable. Because of the importance of extrinsic sugars in the process of dental caries, persistent and long standing use of syrupy medication is of particular concern in children with chronic illness[1], and any sector of the population who are dentate. Chronically sick children who suffer from, or need to be protected from, frequent infections are more at risk. Drug companies are responding, albeit slowly, to the demand for 'sugar-free' medicines, and whenever possible, the dental profession encourages the prescription of sugar-free or artificially sweetened substitutes.

8.3 Contact reactions

Toxic reactions may occur as a result of direct contact between medication and the delicate oral soft tissues. If drugs are allowed to pool in the mouth, an inflammatory reaction may occur. In older persons with thin and atrophic oral soft tissues, the reaction may be severe. Large ulcerated areas in the floor of the mouth are sometimes caused by medicine or tablets which have not been swallowed. By observing whether medication has been swallowed, it may be possible to prevent this potential complication.

Chemical burns occur due to prolonged contact of drugs with oral tissues. The practice of using aspirin or alcohol in direct contact with a painful tooth can lead to chemical burns which may be more painful than the condition they were used to relieve (*Colour Plate* **19**). Patients should be advised to comply with the use of medication as indicated on the package.

8.4 Drugs in pregnancy

It is well accepted that medication during pregnancy is best avoided, particularly during the first three months. In the case of drugs which are found to affect the development of the foetus (teratogens), the facial structures, including jaws and teeth, may also be affected. The degree of abnormality depends upon the dose and stage of foetal development at which the drug is given.

Certain drugs should be avoided during the period of tooth development. Tetracycline and its derivatives cause discoloration within the developing tooth structure; teeth may have an overall blue tinge. This is not damaging to the tooth structure, but may be cosmetically unacceptable.

8.5 Oral side-effects

Although the oral side-effects of drugs are relatively uncommon, it is worth noting the preparations which may be prescribed for the treatment of conditions covered in Section 3. In some cases, oral infection and ulceration are secondary to drug-induced blood disorders. Drugs which reduce salivary secretions have the potential to increase the rate of caries and periodontal disease and increase the risk of oral infection and other lesions.

Oral Effects of Medication

The frequency of side-effects is variable and will be affected by the individual's state of health and interactions with other drugs and treatments. Drugs which may be abused are also included in this section. Possible side-effects are summarised in *Table 8.1*, although the list is by no means comprehensive.

8.6 Summary

A comprehensive account of the oral side-effects of medication is beyond the scope of this guide. Interactions between drugs are even more complex, and with the number of new drugs available each year the section would become rapidly out of date. However, it is important for health professionals to be aware of the potential for oral side-effects, particularly sugar in medicines and dry mouth, and the implications for oral health.

We suggest that the reader refers to the most recent issue of the *British National Formulary*[2], which is published twice a year, to obtain up-to-date information on possible side-effects. Suspected adverse drug reactions should be reported to the Committee on the Safety of Medicines on the Yellow Card. Health care professionals should be aware of the reporting system described in the British National Formulary.

8.7 References

1. Hobson, P. *et al.* (1987). Sugar-based medicines and dental disease – progress report. *Community Dental Health*, **4**(2), 169–176.
2. *British National Formulary.* (1991) London, British Medical Association and Royal Pharmaceutical Society of Great Britain.

Table 8.1 Oral side-effects of different medications

Side-effects	Drugs
Dry mouth	Amphetamines Antihistamines Antihypertensives Anti-Parkinsonian drugs Appetite suppressants Atropine and its derivatives Bronchodilators Decongestants Ganglion-blocking agents Lithium Monoamine oxidase inhibitors Phenothiazines Propantheline Tricyclic antidepressants
Oral infections	Broad-spectrum antibiotics Corticosteroids Cytotoxics Immunosuppressives Drugs which cause dry mouth
Ulceration	Cocaine Cytotoxics Gold Indomethacin Isoprenaline Penicillamine Phenylbutazone Potassium chloride
Gingival swelling	Cyclosporin (*Colour Plate* **20**) Diltiazem Nifedipine (*Colour Plate* **18**) Phenytoin (*Colour Plate* **17**)
Blistered areas	Busulphan Captopril Carbamazepine Clonidine Frusemide Penicillamine Phenylbutazone
Involuntary facial movements	Butyrophenones Carbamazepine L-dopa Methyldopa Metoclopramide Phenothiazines Tetrabenazine Tricyclic antidepressants

(*continued*)

Table 8.1 Oral side-effects of different medications (*continued*)

Side-effects	Drugs
Tooth discoloration	
Superficial staining	Chlorhexidine
	Iron
Developmental discoloration	Fluoride
	Tetracycline

9 Aids to Oral Self-Care, Rehabilitation and Independence

9.1 Introduction
9.2 Environmental factors
9.3 Detection of plaque
9.4 Toothbrushes
9.5 Dental floss and flossing tapes
9.6 Interdental brushes
9.7 Oral irrigation devices
9.8 Other oral hygiene aids
9.9 Toothpastes
9.10 Fluorides
9.11 Mouthwashes and other preparations
9.12 Saliva substitutes
9.13 Adaptations
9.14 Mouth appliances for independence
9.15 Summary
9.16 References

9.1 Introduction

This chapter describes and summarises aids to oral health currently available. Advice is given on adaptations for people with manual and other forms of disability which affect the individual's ability to be self-caring. Although individual oral hygiene advice lies within the remit of the dental hygienist, it is felt this chapter will be of particular interest to a wider audience as it also covers mouthpieces for independence.

9.2 Environmental factors

Environmental factors which have been covered in Chapter 7 fall within the remit of several disciplines. Advice on the design of the physical environment to facilitate independence may be obtained from Independent Living Centres (Appendix 2).

Aids to Self-Care, Rehabilitation and Independence

9.3 Detection of plaque

Before considering the various tools for oral health, it is helpful to visibly identify areas where plaque accumulates. Plaque is normally invisible except in the neglected mouth; disclosing materials dye plaque, identifying areas which have been missed or require extra attention. They are useful for training and monitoring toothbrushing skills and enable the individual or carer to identify areas which require extra attention.

Both tablets and solutions are available. A food dye forms an effective substitute for disclosing solutions provided the individual is not at risk of food allergies. Tablets are unsuitable for individuals with oral dysfunction or inability to comply. For these individuals, solutions which can be painted or swabbed may be more useful for the carer to identify areas of plaque; they can be applied with a cotton bud or swab.

9.4 Toothbrushes

It is universally accepted in the dental literature that the most effective tool for mouthcare is a toothbrush. The nursing profession in evaluating tools currently in use are in general agreement that toothbrushes are superior to traditional methods of oral care with foam sticks, swabbing or topical swab and forceps.[1-8] A child's toothbrush is reported to be more comfortable[1], easier to manipulate and less traumatic if correctly used[2] and yet in the authors' experience, hospital toothbrushes are issued in a standard size with cost being a prime factor in the selection of brand. Different types of toothbrush are described in this section.

Manual toothbrushes

These come in all shapes and sizes (*Figure 2.4*). The most suitable is a small-headed brush with medium to soft filaments – with the proviso that it is replaced as soon as the filaments start to splay at the end. A recently marketed brand has coloured filaments which lose their colour with wear, providing a visual reminder that the toothbrush should be replaced.

Variations in the shank, handle and angle of the head provide a wide choice for the self-caring. Children require a smaller head than adults. The handle of one brand can be bent by heating in hot water, a useful feature when the angle of head to handle needs to be modified. Another is useful for hospital care as it can be autoclaved.

A double-headed toothbrush (*Figure 9.1*) which permits simultaneous brushing of both palatal or lingual and buccal surfaces of the teeth has been shown to be effective, as the bristles are angulated to contact the gingival margins at the correct angle.[9] The handle can be adjusted by immersing it in hot water and bending to the required position. This may be useful for

Holistic Oral Care

Figure 9.1 Double-headed toothbrush

Figure 9.2 Single-tufted toothbrush

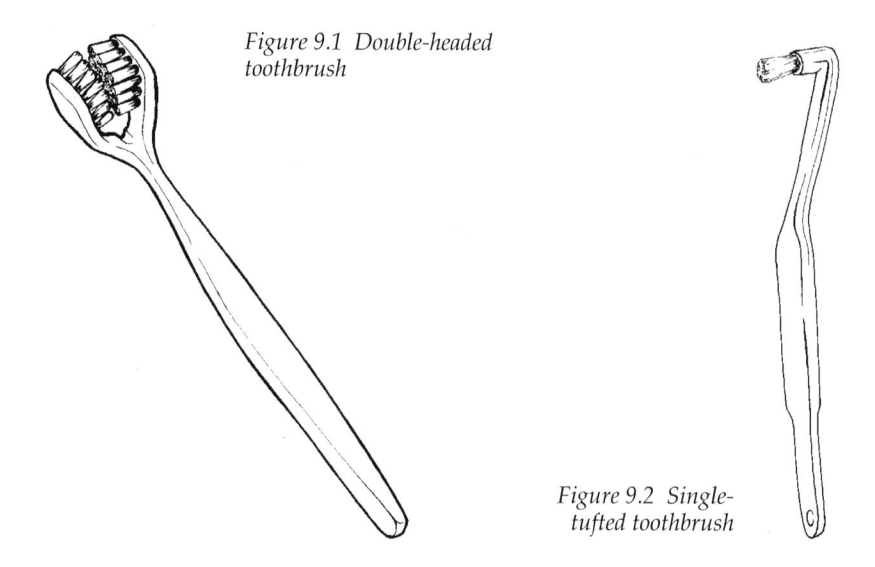

some disabled individuals who find that toothbrushing is tiring, as both outer and inner surfaces are being brushed at the same time. A conventional toothbrush would still be required for occlusal surfaces.

Electric toothbrushes

There are a range of models which are mains operated, rechargeable or battery operated. They are significantly heavier and have a wide handle with small replacement toothbrush heads. Brush head movement varies in different models, however the universal principle is that the brush is held in contact with each site for a specific period of time. All surfaces should be covered systematically without applying excess pressure.

Electric toothbrushes are thought to be useful for disabled people. They are no more or less efficient than good manual toothbrushing, and if used for too short a period give a false sense of oral cleanliness; this is particularly true of battery-operated models, which lose their charge and thus their efficiency over a period of time.

They may be useful for people with reduced manual dexterity or limited wrist movement and for those who lack the cognitive skills to learn the perceptuo-motor skills required to render the mouth plaque free. The wide handle may be advantageous where grip is restricted but the total weight may be a disadvantage. They may well have gimmick value in encouraging compliance and seem to be well tolerated by children and those dependent for oral care. However, investment in what may be an expensive appliance for people who are likely to be on a low income should follow advice from the dental hygienist to ensure that the most suitable model is purchased and that it will be used correctly. Practical instruction may be required.

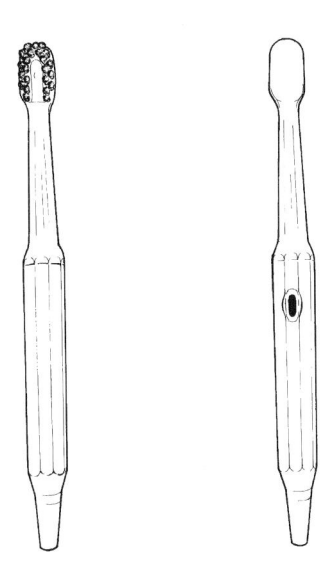

Aids to Self-Care, Rehabilitation and Independence

Figure 9.3 The toothbrush is hollow and the end fits directly onto the aspirator tubing. By covering the hole in the handle of the toothbrush, suction can be varied.

Single-tufted toothbrushes

Variations in brush heads are designed for reaching difficult areas, e.g. for removing plaque from spaces between teeth, around crowns or bridges and malpositioned teeth, and around fixed orthodontic appliances. They are designed to reach areas which other brushes do not reach and should be used with a circular action (*Figure 9.2*).

Aspirating toothbrush

This is useful for the dependent or dysphagic patient in a nursing setting with an aspirator on site (*Figure 9.3*). Maintaining oral health is difficult; care must be taken to protect the airway and since toothbrushing may stimulate salivary flow and create frothing, integral aspiration has obvious benefits. It is useful where vision is restricted and to ensure that toothpaste does not remain in the mouth since toothpaste has a drying effect. An ordinary toothbrush can be modified for use with an aspirator. The central bristles are cut away and a fine Ryle's tube strapped to the handle and tied firmly to the head; however, it is not as efficient as the commercial product.

9.5 Dental floss and flossing tapes

Plaque is not removed from interproximal areas (*Figure 1.3*) by brushing. There are a large number of brands of floss and tape which have different features and claims by manufacturers.

Dental floss is a fine cord which is sometimes waxed and/or flavoured and usually sold on a reel with an integral dispenser. Waxed

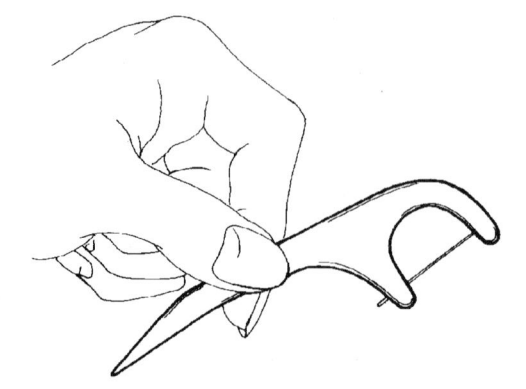

Figure 9.4 Floss holder: the handle can be extended or enlarged to improve the grip.

floss is less likely to catch or tear on rough or defective tooth surfaces, while unwaxed floss separates into several strands, providing more friction and, being finer, passes between the teeth more easily. A new flossing product on the UK market consists of strips of elasticated tape – the rationale being that it is easier to use, provides greater friction and is less likely to catch on fillings. Floss used incorrectly can damage the gingival tissues and over time may saw into the tooth structure. It therefore requires skill and manual dexterity to be used correctly (*Figure 2.3*).

It is extremely difficult if not impossible to handle dental floss if dexterity is impaired. A floss holder (*Figure 9.4*) is available which may overcome some of the difficulties; the handles may need to be enlarged to ensure adequate grip. Some have to be threaded each time they are used; others with floss already attached are for single use. A floss holder which has a longer handle has recently appeared on the UK market and appears to have more potential for people with restricted manual skills.

9.6 Interdental brushes

These are small fine tapered bristle brushes, shaped like the old-fashioned bottle brush, used to remove plaque from crevices and between the roots of teeth (*Figure 9.5*). They can be mounted on the end of a specialised toothbrush handle or hand held; the latter is difficult for people with impaired dexterity.

9.7 Oral irrigation devices

Irrigation devices are designed to flush out food and debris and reduce the concentration of bacterial plaque. Simple versions include rubber-bulbed and metal syringes. Commercial devices are electrically controlled with a

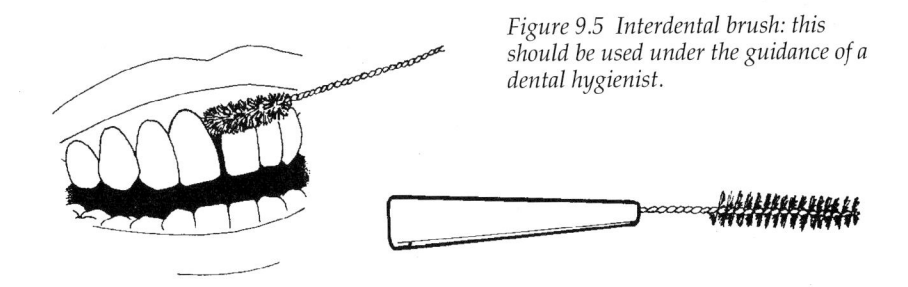

Aids to Self-Care, Rehabilitation and Independence

Figure 9.5 Interdental brush: this should be used under the guidance of a dental hygienist.

water reservoir or are water-driven and attached directly to a water supply. They provide a pulsating jet for irrigation. Some models have the facility to deliver antibacterial agents. They have greater cleansing efficiency and are claimed to stimulate gingival tissue.

They are useful for cleansing around fixed orthodontic appliances, wire fixation and other fixed appliances. Disabled and dependent patients may benefit from their use provided that the airway is not compromised. They should not however be used on patients who are at risk of bacteraemia. Irrigation devices with detachable heads which can be sterilised are valuable aids to oral hygiene in hospital care.

9.8 Other oral hygiene aids

These include gauze strips and pipe cleaners for cleaning wider gaps between teeth, wood sticks and toothpicks, rubber- and plastic-tipped devices. Care should be taken in using some of these devices as they may cause trauma if used incorrectly; their use is recommended under the guidance of a hygienist.

Mouth packs containing foam sticks which are expensive and ineffective except when toothbrushing is impossible are no substitute for gentle toothbrushing.[2,3,10] As awareness of oral health increases, so new oral hygiene products appear on the market; professional advice should be got before purchasing new and relatively expensive oral hygiene aids.

9.9 Toothpastes

For the dental profession the main purpose of toothpaste is as a means of delivering fluoride and other therapeutic substances to the teeth and soft tissues and as a motivator to plaque removal. The potential cosmetic and cleansing sensation may be of greater importance to the user, however. It is important to remove toothpaste after brushing because of the drying effect.

The preventive importance of fluoride in toothpaste has been discussed in Chapters 1–3. Manufacturers' claims for plaque inhibition, tartar control and desensitisation can be confirmed in the United Kingdom by the presence of the British Dental Association's logo on the package. Toothpastes which contain hexetidine have been demonstrated to reduce salivary bacteria, although less effectively than 1% chlorhexidine gluconate gel.[11]

9.10 Fluorides

Dietary fluoride supplements are covered in Chapters 2 and 3 (*Table 2.4*). Tablets are only recommended for systemic use in childhood and early teens, during the period of developing dentition.

Self-applied topical fluorides are available as a rinse, a gel for tray application and a brush-on gel. Supervision may be necessary to ensure that fluoride rinse is retained in the mouth for 1 minute and then expectorated. Professional advice on the most suitable concentration and method is advisable.

Sodium fluoride, available as a 2% solution diluted for daily and weekly rinsing, is also available ready diluted to 0.05% for weekly use; it is fairly well tolerated. It is suggested that stannous fluoride is more effective in caries reduction than sodium fluoride[12], but it has an astringent taste, may cause gingival irritation, and is more likely to stain teeth.[13] Stannous fluoride, which is also available as a 4% gel for brushing, is useful if the correct procedure for rinsing cannot be carried out.

Neutral pH fluoride preparations of 0.5–1% are more easily tolerated by patients who have received radiation treatment[14], although 0.4% stannous fluoride gel administered in a tray is recommended for radiation caries following bone marrow transplants.[15]

Subjective assessment should be a factor in selecting the most suitable topical fluoride regime for individuals who find that fluoride rinsing is painful or have difficulty with compliance. Topical fluorides are of particular importance for adults at risk of dental caries and it is important to ensure a suitable regime by obtaining professional advice.

9.11 Mouthwashes and other preparations

Mouthwashes facilitate the removal of debris, lubricate tissues, and in some cases have antibacterial or antiseptic properties. Many of the proprietary products currently available which claim to have specific oral benefits should not be toxic to oral tissues.[16] A commonly advertised mouthwash contains a high proportion of alcohol, which in the compromised

Aids to Self-Care, Rehabilitation and Independence

patient may be toxic to oral tissue and exacerbate the oral condition. Agents currently in common usage are summarised below.

Chlorhexidine gluconate

Chlorhexidine gluconate is a chemical anti-plaque agent also available as a gel and spray. Although it has the disadvantage of staining teeth, staining is reversible and easily removed professionally. It may produce mucosal irritation in rare cases. However, its demonstrated effectiveness against plaque[17] far outweighs these side-effects. It is available in two flavours, normal and mint, although complaints have been made about the taste.[18]

Mouthrinses may be unsuitable for certain disabled groups; clinical trials with chlorhexidine gluconate 1% administered as a gel in splints to a group of subjects with learning difficulties demonstrated a reduction in bacterial plaque.[19] Chlorhexidine gluconate 1% administered as a spray was preferred to both mouthwash and gel by parents and carers of a group of children with cerebral palsy[20]; it was less effective than the gel – nevertheless, willingness to comply with this method is an important factor.[21] Chlorhexidine spray offers a long overdue solution to chemical plaque control in patients who may be unable to co-operate with brushing or rinsing.

There is ample evidence of the effectiveness of chlorhexidine gluconate in bacterial plaque reduction.[17] It is recommended as an aid to mechanical cleansing in the initial oral hygiene phase of treatment. Recommendations for its use when mechanical oral hygiene is difficult are summarised in *Table 9.1*.

Table 9.1 Chlorhexidine: recommendations for use.

- Post oral surgery
- Fixation of the jaws
- Fixed orthodontic appliances
- People whose oral health may be affected by disability
- Medically compromised and systemic diseases affecting the oral tissues

Hexetidine

Hexetidine 1% is marketed as a mouthwash and gargle. It is similar to chlorhexidine but has less anti-plaque effect at 1% concentration than the latter.[22] There has been very little research on this agent.

Cetylpyridinium chloride

This is also marketed as a mouthwash or gargle which contains 0.05% cetylpyridinium chloride. It has a moderate anti-plaque effect against gram-positive bacteria, however it is not as effective as chlorhexidine.[16,23]

Oxygenating agents

These include hydrogen peroxide and sodium perborate. They have a mechanical cleansing effect due to frothing in contact with oral debris. Their mucosolvent properties may be useful in breaking down thick and viscous saliva, however they are not recommended for long-term use.

Hydrogen peroxide 3% (10 volume) diluted as a mouth wash has an unpleasant taste[18] and is modestly antiseptic. It should be used with caution since it may cause chemical burns if incorrectly diluted. It may be unsuitable for patients with stomatitis whose oral mucosa is at risk of providing entry for systemic infection since it breaks down normal tissue[18]. However a dilute aqueous solution of 3% hydrogen peroxide and sodium bicarbonate is reported to decrease bacterial activity and alleviate salivary acidity in patients with bone marrow transplants[24].

Sodium perborate has similar properties to hydrogen peroxide, may be caustic if inadequately diluted, and there is a risk of borate toxicity due to absorption. It is contraindicated for children under 5 years and in patients suffering from renal insufficiency, and it should not be used for longer than 7 days.

Sodium bicarbonate

Sodium bicarbonate has mucosolvent properties and an unpleasant taste. It is frequently cited in nursing literature but there is little evidence to confirm its usefulness other than as a cleansing agent. Dudjak[25] reports that sodium bicarbonate was perceived as providing a lower perception of oral comfort than hydrogen peroxide. Further research is necessary to identify its usefulness.

Phenol

This is available for use as a throat spray or diluted as a gargle or mouthwash. Epiglottis and laryngeal oedema have been reported to the Committee on the Safety of Medicines and it is therefore contraindicated in patients with epiglottitis and for children.[26] There has been inadequate research to assess the effect of phenol on bacterial plaque[17].

Povidone iodine

There is little information on povidone iodine 1% which, although it is recommended for use as a gargle or mouthwash, appears to have no anti-plaque activity at this dilution[17]. Reported side-effects include mucosal irritation and hypersensitivity reactions.

Thymol

Thymol and its derivatives are used in mouthwashes at relatively high concentrations, at which anti-bacterial activity has been reported.[17] Thymol

Aids to Self-Care, Rehabilitation and Independence

glycerine is reported to be initially refreshing.[1] Although glycerine acts as a lubricant, its astringent effect is a contraindication in patients with xerostomia (dry mouth). Thymol preparations do not appear to offer any advantage over mouthwashes demonstrated to be effective antibacterial agents at lower concentrations.

Sodium chloride
Isotonic saline is effective and well tolerated as a mechanical cleansing agent. A warm solution is recommended in the management of mucositis (Chapter 15). Sodium chloride mouthwash Co. BP contains 1% sodium chloride and 1.5% sodium bicarbonate with flavouring and chloroform water; although this may be more palatable, there is little evidence to suggest that it has any advantage over normal saline.

Benzydamine hydrochloride
This is reported to be effective for the relief of oral ulceration. It is available as a rinse or spray; occasional numbness or stinging are reported side-effects.

Other preparations
Lemon and glycerine swabs continue to be used in the nursing setting. Their usefulness is questionable[27]; glycerine although lubricating, is astringent, and lemon stimulates salivary secretion.[1] Overuse may lead to exhaustion of the salivary glands and increased xerostomia. The low pH increases the risk of dental caries. Other common oral preparations may contain alcohol. They have no demonstrable benefits over known anti-plaque agents and are contraindicated in patients with alcohol abuse. Tap water is a cheap and effective substitute in the absence of professional advice, while chlorhexidine gluconate is currently the most effective chemical anti-plaque agent.

9.12 Saliva substitutes

Water, ice chips and atomised water sprays are simple and provide relief. Proprietary saliva substitutes are, however, necessary for chronic xerostomia, particularly for radiation xerostomia.

Hypromellose, which acts as a lubricant, can be obtained without the additional substances included in Artificial Saliva DPF. Other proprietary products include Glandosane, Luborant and Saliva Orthana. Glandosane is delivered by spraying onto the oral mucosa. Luborant, also delivered by spray, contains fluoride. Saliva Orthana is expensive and available for hospital use only; it contains gastric mucin and is recommended for radiation xerostomia and other conditions that produce severe xerostomia.

Holistic Oral Care

9.13 Adaptations

Disability and impaired manual dexterity may lead to a deterioration in self care. Inability to grip, stiff joints, limited arm movement and reduced control may restrict oral care using conventional oral hygiene aids. A simple adaptation may be all that is required to enable the individual to manage their own oral care. A number of cheap and simple devices are described and illustrated. Liaison between occupational therapist and hygienist may be necessary to ensure correctly adapted tools. A list of useful aids to oral hygiene can be obtained from the Disabled Living Foundation.[28]

Toothbrushing aids

Enlarged handles improve grip. Adaptations can be constructed from cheap and readily available items (*Figures 9.6, 9.7*).

Epoxy resin and thermoplastic materials can be used to adapt toothbrush handles in cases of manual deformity (*Figure 9.8*). AHRTAG produce a leaflet illustrating a range of individual adaptations and their uses.[29] More expensive proprietary aids can be used to hold oral hygiene aids as well as items such as cutlery, pens, etc.

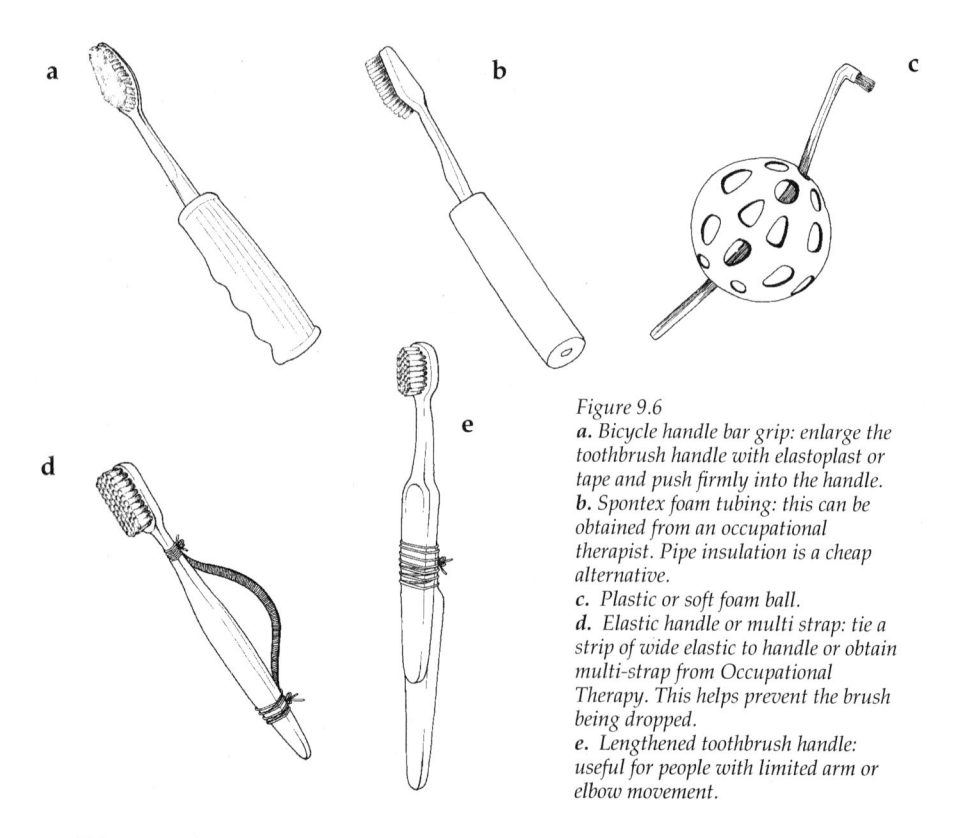

Figure 9.6
a. Bicycle handle bar grip: enlarge the toothbrush handle with elastoplast or tape and push firmly into the handle.
b. Spontex foam tubing: this can be obtained from an occupational therapist. Pipe insulation is a cheap alternative.
c. Plastic or soft foam ball.
d. Elastic handle or multi strap: tie a strip of wide elastic to handle or obtain multi-strap from Occupational Therapy. This helps prevent the brush being dropped.
e. Lengthened toothbrush handle: useful for people with limited arm or elbow movement.

Aids to Self-Care, Rehabilitation and Independence

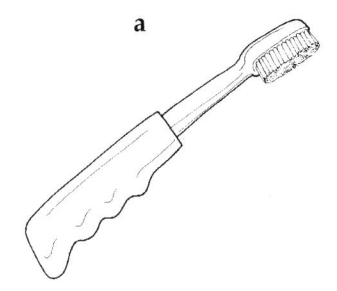

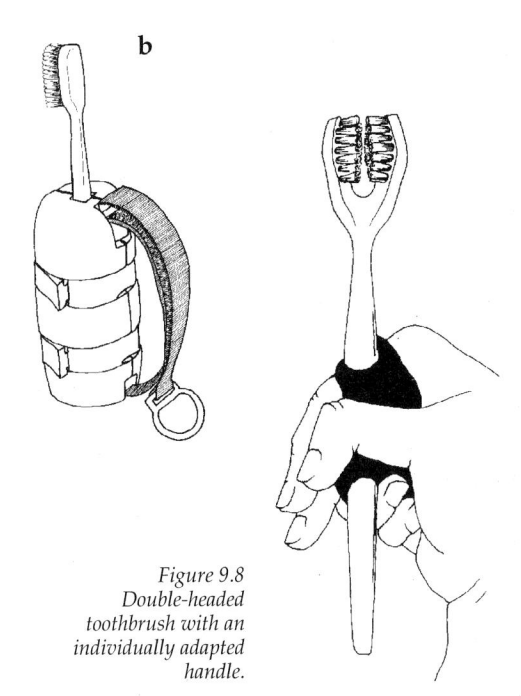

Figure 9.7
a. *Commercially produced aid to gripping and holding, designed for handling cutlery.*
b. *Gripmate: a more expensive aid which can also be used to assist with holding pen, cutlery etc. The strap prevents it being dropped and the device has a number of openings for gripping items in different positions.*

*Figure 9.8
Double-headed toothbrush with an individually adapted handle.*

Straps help to prevent the brush from being dropped. Long-handled holders which accept a toothbrush extend the reach of individuals with stiff or limited arm movements; a simple device can be made by lengthening the handle with a wooden splint. Occupational therapies will advise and stock a wide range of adaptations for specific manual problems, including splints and arm supports.

A wall-mounted toothbrush holder individually constructed may be of benefit in helping the tetraplegic individual to maintain some control over personal care.[28,30] It should not be relied on to provide effective oral hygiene without individual assessment and support from a hygienist.

Denture cleaning aids
Loss of use of one hand can be frustrating for denture care, which normally requires two hands. Denture brushes which stick to the sink with rubber suction cups help to overcome this problem. An ordinary nail brush can be adapted by screwing suction cups to the back; proprietary products are also available with suction cups attached and a variety of brush heads (*Figure 9.9, 9.10*).

Other aids
Pump-operated toothpaste dispensers, self-pasting toothbrushes and tube squeezers may overcome problems of using oral hygiene materials. A safety pin through the cap of the tube enables the individual with limited

Holistic Oral Care

Figure 9.9 Commercial denture brushes
a. *Wide handled denture brush for improved grip, with two brushing heads.*
b. *As **a**, but with three brushing heads and suction cups for attaching firmly to sink.*

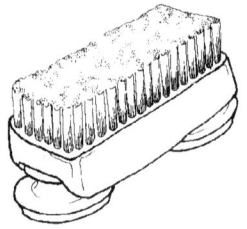

Figure 9.10 Nail brush adapted for cleaning dentures: suction cups have been screwed to the back of an ordinary nailbrush to secure it firmly to the sink.

grip to unscrew the cap. Beakers with lids, lips or handles and straws may assist with rinsing and the use of mouthwashes or fluorides. The Pat Saunders drinking straw has a non-returnable valve for individuals with difficulty in sucking. It requires just a little imagination to design a simple aid or adapt an appliance to overcome many day-to-day problems; the occupational therapist and hygienist can advise on specific problems. Disabled Living Centres provide a useful source of advice for aids which facilitate oral self-care (Appendix 2).

9.14 Mouth appliances for independence

People with severely impaired movement of the upper limbs may benefit from mouth-held devices which enable them to communicate or control environmental controls and computer systems, paint, operate lathes and all manner of equipment. Mouthpieces are individually designed and involve the occupational therapist at initial assessment and on completion to ensure the aid is appropriate and to provide suitable end-pieces for the individual's needs.

Mouthpieces consist of a splint which fits over the teeth and to which various tools may be attached.[31-33] A mouthpiece which is attached to a partial denture has been constructed, enabling a multiple sclerosis sufferer with hand tremor to write and paint.[34] Tongue-controlled switches fitted to the palatal surfaces of a mouthpiece have been designed to control an electric wheelchair[35]. Natural healthy teeth are an advantage in designing a stable and successful mouth-controlled appliance. Oral health needs to be regularly monitored to ensure that mouthpieces do not damage oral tissues. The dental team can make a significant contribution to rehabilitation and independence for people with disabilities.

9.15 Summary

This chapter summarises information on various oral hygiene aids. It includes aids to maintain oral health and independence. The self-caring individual who attends routinely has easy access to individual oral hygiene advice from the dental team. For those with a special need, oral and dental assessment will identify specific need areas which can be addressed. A home visit should be requested for the disabled and housebound to obtain appropriate advice. The dental hygienist and the occupational therapist, who together provide domiciliary care and advice under the National Health Service in the UK, can monitor the use and effectiveness of these aids.

9.16 References

1. Howarth, H. (1977). Mouthcare procedures for the very ill, *Nursing Times*, **73**, 10, 354–355.
2. Shepherd, G., Page, C. and Sammon, P. (1987). Oral hygiene, *Nursing Times*, **83**, 19, 25–27.
3. Harris, M.D. (1980). Tools for mouthcare, *Nursing Times*, **76**, 8, 340–342.
4. Miller, R. and Rubenstein, L. (1987). Oral health for hospitalised patients: The nurse's role, *Journal of Nursing Education*, **26**, 9, 362–366.
5. Watson, R. (1989). Care of the mouth, *Nursing*, **3**, 44, 20–24.
6. Lewis, I. (1984). Developing a research-based curriculum: An exercise in relation to oral care, *Nurse Education Today*, **3**, 6, 143–144.
7. Allbright, A. (1984). Oral care for the cancer chemotherapy patient, *Nursing Times*, **80**, 21, 40–42.
8. Trenter, P. and Creason, N. (1986). Nurse-administered oral hygiene. Is there a scientific basis?, *Journal of Advanced Nursing*, **11**, 3, 323–331.
9. Agerholm, D.M. (1991). A clinical trial to evaluate plaque removal with a double-headed toothbrush, *Brit. Dent. J.*, **170**, 411–413.
10. Sullivan, M. and Fleming, T. (1986). Oral care for the radiotherapy treated head and neck cancer patient, *Dental Hygiene*, **60**, 3, 112.
11. Moran, J., Addy, M. and Newcombe, R. (1988). The antibacterial effect of toothpastes on the salivary flora, *Jour. Clin. Periodont.*, **15**, 193.
12. Forrest, J.O. (1987). Stannous fluoride gel in preventive practice, *Dental Practice*, March 5, 13.

13. Cawson, R.A. and Spector, R.G. (1989). Antiseptics, anti-caries agents and related drugs used in routine dentistry, in *Clinical Pharmacology in Dentistry*, 5th ed., Churchill Livingstone, Edinburgh, p. 53.
14. Rothwell, B.R. (1987). Prevention and treatment of the orofacial complications of radiotherapy, *Jour. Am. Dent. Ass.*, **114**, 316–322.
15. Maxymiw, W.G. and Wood, R.E. (1989). The role of dentistry in patients undergoing bone marrow transplantation, *Br. Dent. J.*, **167**, 229–234.
16. Hogg, S. (1990). Chemical Control of Plaque, *Dental Update*, Oct, 330–334.
17. Addy, M. (1986). Chlorhexidine compared with other locally delivered microbials: a short review, *J. Clin. Periodonol.*, **13**, 957–964.
18. Pritchard, A.P. and David, J.A. (Ed) (1988). *The Royal Marsden Hospital Manual of Clinical Nursing Procedures*, 2nd ed., London, Harper and Row.
19. Storhaug, K. (1977). Hibitane in oral disease in handicapped patients, *J. Clin. Periodontol.*, **4**, 102.
20. Francis, J.R., Addy, M. and Hunter, B. (1987). A comparison of three delivery methods of chlorhexidine in handicapped children. Part II. Parent and houseparent preferences, *J. Periodontol.*, **58**, 7, 456–459.
21. Francis, J.R., Hunter, B. and Addy, M. (1987). A comparison of three delivery methods of chlorhexidine in handicapped children, Part I. Effect on plaque gingivitis and tooth staining, *J. Periodontol.*, **58**, 7, 451–455.
22. Cawson. R.A. and Spector, R.G. (1989). Antiseptics, anticaries agents and related drugs used in dentistry, in *Clinical Pharmacology in Dentistry*, 5th ed., Churchill Livingstone, Edinburgh, p. 58.
23. Volpe, A.R. *et al.* (1969). Antimicrobial control of bacterial plaque and calculus, and the effects of these agents on oral flora, *J. Dent. Research*, **48**, 832–841.
24. Carl, W and Higby, P. (1985). Oral manifestations of bone marrow transplantation, *Clin. Oncol.*, **8**, 81–87.
25. Dudjak, L.A. (1987). Mouth care for mucositis due to radiation therapy, *Cancer Nursing*, **10**, 3, 131–139.
26. *British National Formulary*. (1991) London, British Medical Association and Royal Pharmaceutical Society of Great Britain.
27. Barnett, J. (1991). A reassessment of oral healthcare, *Prof. Nurse*, Sept., 703–708.
28. *Dentistry and Disability: notes for disabled people and non-dental professionals*, (1987). Disabled Living Foundation Information Service, London.
29. Caston, D. (1981). *How to Make Handgrips*, London, Appropriate Health Resources and Technologies Action Group.
30. Spratley, M.H. (1991). A toothbrushing aid for a quadriplegic patient, *Spec. Care Dent.*, **11**, 3, 114–115.
31. Kozole, K.P *et al.* (1985), Modular mouthstick system, *Journ. Pros. Dent.*, **53**, 6, 831–835.
32. Warren, K. (1990). Mouthstick prostheses and other gadgets, *Dental Update*, Dec., 428, 430.
33. O'Donnel, D., Yenn, P.K.J. and Robinson, W. (1985). A mouth-controlled appliance for severely physically handicapped patients, *Br. Dent. J.*, 159, 186–188.
34. Garsrud, O. (1981). Therapeutic dental aid for patient with multiple sclerosis, *Brit. Dent. J.*, **150**, 356.
35. Barker, C.B. (1981). A linguo-buccal aid to control an electric wheelchair, *Brit. Dent. J.*, Oct., 263–264.

Section 3

At-Risk Groups: People with a Special Need

Introduction to Section 3

There are certain groups, which due to illness or treatment, disability, handicap or lifestyle, are more at risk of oral and dental disease from the barriers that they may experience. The increased risks can be summarised under three headings:

- Access.
- Attitude.
- Ability.

Access

Access has two aspects: access to information, and access to services.

Access to information
Section 3 will provide information in depth on specific oral and dental problems. It is anticipated that making this information accessible to healthcare professionals and their patients will increase an individual's access to information, relevant to his or her particular situation.

Access to services
A mobility handicap leads to social isolation, which is itself a barrier to obtaining information, and conditions people over the years to have a very low expectation of services. Disabled people consistently quote access – to information, transport systems and buildings – as the key to independence and choice.

In a case for anti-discrimination legislation, Barnes[1] points out that the physical environment of mainstream housing, transport and the architectural infrastructure has been constructed without reference to the needs of disabled people. The lack of accessibility of Health Authority premises is highlighted in a survey of services for people with a physical disability.[2]

Chapter 5 on Dental Services and the Dental Team provided the framework for seeking appropriate advice and dental care. Information on physical access and associated problems, such as the availability of suitable transport systems, should be made easily available in each district. The development of Social Care Plans and the increasing co-operation between Health and Social Services may help to provide a more comprehensive information source. As yet there is no statutory body with the responsibility for such a role.

At-Risk Groups: People with a Special Need

Attitudes

Attitudes to oral health and disease, to the need for oral care, regular dental attendance, and the relative value placed on these factors in the context of the individual's illness or disability, underpin this guide. We hope this section will help change professional attitudes to the value and importance of oral health in holistic care.

Ability

Ability includes the individual's physical and cognitive abilities to carry out effective oral care and to seek dental services. It also includes the ability of carers, whether family, informal or professional, to provide advice and care for those who are dependent on them for personal needs or require assistance.

In referring to dependence for oral care, we do not mean the dependency created by institutional practices. We accept the arguments of disabled people that dependence is not an intrinsic feature of impairment and disability but is socially created by a disabling and disablist society[3].

Although the chapter headings partly follow medical diagnostic patterns, the contents are arranged to cover similar oral problems and the management of oral care. For example, cerebral palsy is covered in depth in Chapter 10 on physical disability and sensory impairment, with a small section in Chapter 11 on people with learning disabilities. Epilepsy, which is a symptom of a neurological disorder, is included in Chapter 10, although it is a relatively common symptom in conditions associated with brain damage, whether congenital or acquired. Epilepsy is also discussed in Chapters 11 and 12.

There will inevitably be some overlap between chapters because illness and disability are multifactorial. The essence of quality care lies in accurate assessment of the individual, and it may be necessary to dip into several chapters to find all the relevant information.

In conclusion, in 1988, at an international conference on oral health and disability, Justin Dart[4], Chairperson of the United States Congressional Task Force on the Rights and Empowerment of Americans with Disabilities, stated:

> *Quality dental care contributes to basic health and to the development of the type of self-image and social image that will be absolutely essential for the emergence of people with disabilities from an eternity of oppression.*

We do not have such grandiose expectations for this guide, but we do hope that this section in particular will give the professional the necessary information to enable people with disability or illness to improve their oral health, as a contribution to holistic health and health gain.[5]

References

1. Barnes, C. (1991). Housing, transport and the built environment. In: *Disabled People in Britain and Discrimination: A Case for Anti-Discrimination Legislation*. London: Hurst and Co., with BCODP.
2. Edwards, F.C. and Warren, M.D. (1990). *Health services for adults with physical disabilities. A survey of District Health Authorities 1988/89*. London: The Royal College of Physicians.
3. Oliver, M. (1990). Social construction of disability. In: *The Politics of Disablement*. London, Macmillan Education, p. 85
4. Dart, J. (1988). Ensuring the rights of persons with disabilities. *Spec. Care in Dent.*, Nov–Dec, 245–248.
5. British Dental Association. (1992). *Quality Care for Oral Health*. London, BDA.

10 Physical Disability and Sensory Impairment

10.1 Introduction
10.2 Prevalence of physical disability
10.3 Barriers to oral health
10.4 Arthritis
10.5 Brittle bone disease (osteogenesis imperfecta)
10.6 Rickets and osteomalacia
10.7 Osteoporosis
10.8 Paget's disease (osteitis deformans)
10.9 Muscular dystrophies and myotonic disorders
10.10 Myasthenia gravis
10.11 Motor neurone disease
10.12 Multiple sclerosis
10.13 Guillain-Barré syndrome
10.14 Stroke (cerebrovascular accident)
10.15 Bell's palsy
10.16 Parkinson's disease
10.17 Cleft lip and palate
10.18 Cerebral palsy
10.19 Spina bifida and hydrocephalus
10.20 Spinal injuries and trauma
10.21 Head injury
10.22 Epilepsy
10.23 Sensory impairment
10.24 Summary
10.25 References

10.1 Introduction

This chapter covers the oral care of people who primarily have a physical disability or sensory impairment. It summarises the commoner conditions which may affect manual dexterity, arm control and mobility, i.e. physical disability which may influence oral health. It also includes oral aspects of physically disabling conditions and the oral side-effects of treatment.

10.2 Prevalence of physical disability

Disability affects a varied and diverse section of the population of all ages and all social classes. The 1988 OPCS survey in Britain estimated that there are over six million adults with one or more disabilities, of which some four million have mobility problems.[1] Approximately 2.5 million were estimated to have problems in managing personal care and a similar number had hearing difficulties.

10.3 Barriers to oral health

Information, transport and access are key issues in the political debate about equal rights for people with a disability. Removal of these barriers is seen as a priority in reducing social handicap. Difficulties in finding accessible dental premises may act as a barrier to oral health. Without regular dental attendance, delays in obtaining preventive advice and treatment often lead to crisis management for pain relief.

A survey of health services in District Health Authorities revealed that casualty departments and out-patient clinics were not universally accessible to the unaided wheelchair user.[2] Dental practices are not renowned for being on the ground-floor with ramped entrances and wide automatic doors, although there is no data to confirm this other than reports of disabled people. Twenty-four per cent of a sample of people with long-term health problems or physical disabilities, complained about access to dentists' and opticians' premises, while one determined person reported using 'firemen to get to the dentist'.[3] Dental surgeries in modern health centres are more likely to be accessible. The Family Health Services Authority is best placed to advise on accessible surgeries in general dental practice (Chapter 5).

Arm control and manual disability may affect the individual's ability to manage oral care effectively. Loss or restricted use of the dominant hand will require that new skills be learnt by the less dominant hand. Aids and adaptations which enable the individual to obtain limited compensation for disability may improve oral self-care skills (Chapter 9). Interdisciplinary assessment by an occupational therapist and dental hygienist may be necessary to ensure that appropriate aids are selected.

Developmental abnormalities which affect oral structures may lead to a range of oral problems which place the individual at increased risk of oral and dental disease. Changes affecting oral musculature may affect oral health. Paralysis, muscle weakness and increased muscle tone contribute to a number of oral problems. It is particularly important that preventive programmes and counselling are initiated at birth, or soon after diagnosis, bearing in mind the psychological effects of diagnosis and adjustment to disability on both the individual and their family or 'carers'.

10.4 Arthritis

Arthritis is the commonest physically disabling condition in the UK, and is estimated to affect approximately 20 million people.[4] Pain is a major disabling symptom[5]. Although there are many different forms, osteoarthritis and rheumatoid arthritis are the main causes of arthritic disease.

Osteoarthritis

Osteoarthritis is characterised by breakdown of the joint cartilage and thickening of the bone. It occurs mainly in later life, affecting the load-bearing joints, hips, knees and spine with pain, stiffness and gradual loss of function. Mobility is reduced, although pain and restricted mobility may be treated by surgical joint replacement. Post-operative anticoagulant therapy may affect dental management.

There are no oral symptoms of osteoarthritis, although medication may have oral side-effects. High aspirin dosage for pain relief leads to a bleeding tendency and may cause delayed healing. Non-steroidal anti-inflammatory drugs (NSAIDs), such as indomethacin, may cause oral ulceration. As osteoarthritis is more common in later life, the oral aspects of ageing must be considered and also the limitations imposed by impaired mobility.

Rheumatoid arthritis

Rheumatoid arthritis is an acutely disabling disease which affects all ages with females more frequently affected than males. It has a variable course, but is generally progressive with severe inflammation. Swelling, acute pain and joint deformity usually first affect hands and feet, and later knees, ankles, wrists and elbows. In the active phases, anaemia is common.

Oral ulceration may occur due to anaemia associated with the condition or secondary to drug therapy. Aspirin, steroids, penicillamine, gold, NSAIDs, and antimalarial drugs are used. Iron may be prescribed for anaemia. Possible oral side-effects (Table 10.1) are dose-related and may be worse during acute phases of illness.

Approximately 15% of rheumatoid arthritis sufferers develop Sjögren's syndrome, the symptoms of which are dry mouth and dry eyes. The symptoms of dry mouth (xerostomia), its consequences and treatment, are covered in several chapters. Added complications of drug side-effects and restrictions to oral care posed by manual disability can exacerbate painful and distressing oral symptoms.

When the temporomandibular joint is affected, mouth opening may be limited, affecting oral care and the management of dental treatment. However, pain in this joint affects relatively few sufferers. Involvement of the cervical vertebrae also poses problems for dental management.

Steroid therapy affects the individual's response to stress; an increase in steroid medication is required to cope with potentially stressful situations,

Table 10.1 Oral side-effects of drugs used in arthritis.

Drug	Oral side-effects
Aspirin	Ulceration
	Delayed healing
Corticosteroids	Candidal infection
Penicillamine	Ulceration
	Loss of taste
Gold	White patches
NSAIDs	Ulceration
	White patches
Antimalarials	White patches
Iron	Discoloured teeth

such as dental extractions or even routine dental treatment. Good oral hygiene and relief of dry mouth are essential for the prevention and alleviation of oral discomfort.

Juvenile arthritis

Juvenile rheumatoid arthritis is rare, but severely disabling. It is estimated to affect one in a thousand children in Britain. There are a number of different types, of which Still's disease is one. Approximately half this group develop severe and chronic disability which is more severe than in adults. Oral problems are similar to those in adults, and care must be taken to ensure protection of the young person's teeth. It is therefore important to stress preventive measures at diagnosis.

10.5 Brittle bone disease (osteogenesis imperfecta)

As lay terminology for this rare condition implies, brittle bone disease is a disorder in which bone is extremely fragile and prone to multiple fractures, particularly in childhood. Although these heal rapidly, permanent physical deformity may result from repeated fractures – leading to a range of physical disabilities.

The condition is largely inherited and has a number of genetic variations, which range from mild to severe. It is basically the result of a defect in the collagen fibres forming the infrastructure for bone formation.

Sometimes it is associated with physical problems which affect general health and therefore the management of dental care, e.g. cardiac abnormalities such as mitral or aortic valvular defects, which require antibiotic cover prior to certain types of invasive dental treatment (Chapter 13).

Teeth may be blue or purplish and abnormally translucent due to defects in tooth structure. When teeth are affected, they are inherently weak due to undeveloped dentine (Chapter 1). Teeth are therefore very prone to wear, and by adolescence may have worn to the gum margins. It is essential to provide regular dental care and preventive regimes from birth.

10.6 Rickets and osteomalacia

Rickets is caused by a deficiency of calcium, phosphorus or vitamin D, which leads to a failure in bone formation. It occurs in children, whereas osteomalacia, which is the disease in adults, presents mainly during pregnancy and lactation. Deficiency may be due to a number of factors, and in the Third World is mainly due to dietary deficiency. It had largely vanished in Britain following improvements in socio-economic conditions and diet. However, it is resurfacing amongst immigrants who have suffered from malnutrition and dietary deficiencies related to cultural food practices.

In children, bones are weak, prone to fracture and deformity, whereas in adults, deformity mainly affects the weight-bearing bones. There may be delays in the eruption of teeth, although tooth structure is rarely affected except in severe cases. When the disease is due to a rare syndrome which affects the absorption of vitamin D, dentine calcification is abnormal, increasing the risk of caries and attrition. Dental care is essential to provide appropriate preventive regimes, and sometimes splints may be needed to protect the surfaces of teeth from further wear.

10.7 Osteoporosis

Osteoporosis is caused by long-term calcium or hormone deficiencies, and results in a reduction in the size of bones and in bone calcium content. It mainly affects women after the menopause; calcium supplements and hormone replacement therapy may be the treatment of choice. It is the commonest underlying cause of fractures in the elderly with the obvious potential for a reduction in mobility. Although there are no oral or dental aspects to osteoporosis, the associated problems of ageing are an important consideration.

10.8 Paget's disease (osteitis deformans)

Paget's disease is a fairly common disorder characterised by enlarged bones which are prone to deformity. It mainly appears in older people and predominantly affects males. The cause is unknown, although theories include hormonal imbalance, heredity, arteriosclerosis and a history of syphilis. It is a slowly progressive disease, in which the first complaint may be that hat, shoes or gloves are too small, or dentures are ill-fitting. If facial bones are involved, the upper jaw is more commonly affected than the lower.

The disease poses problems for dental management. Whereas the teeth are not visibly affected, radiographs may reveal resorbed roots or areas of excessive cement deposits around the roots; this makes dental extractions more difficult. In the earlier stages of the disease, excessive bleeding may follow dental extractions, and in later stages, reduced blood supply to the bone increases the risk of post-extraction infection. Surgical extraction, prophylactic antibiotics and haemorrhage control complicate treatment. Dentures which lose their fit may need to be replaced or modified more frequently.

10.9 Muscular dystrophies and myotonic disorders

Although diseases affecting the musculature are relatively uncommon, muscular dystrophy is the most common muscle disease of childhood. It is an inherited disabling condition caused by a gradual breakdown of the muscle fibres, leading to progressive deterioration which ultimately affects mobility. When shoulder muscles are involved, weakness affects arms and hands.

Duchenne type is the most common and the most severe: it only affects boys, with very rare exceptions. Becker type, which is less disabling, progresses more slowly and mobility is less likely to be affected. There are several other rarer forms which are classified by the groups of muscles affected. In myotonic dystrophy, which occurs mainly in adults, facial weakness, speech and swallowing difficulties may occur.

There are no specific oral features, although malocclusions due to widening of the jaw arches may occur; this is caused by the comparatively greater pressure of the tongue in relation to the weakness of lip and cheek muscles. An 'open mouth' posture due to weak facial muscles poses a risk to oral health. This leads to dryness of the oral tissues which, combined with a reduction in oral self-care due to upper limb weakness, increases the risk factors for caries and periodontal disease. Swallowing difficulties may complicate oral care. Medical complications which affect dental management include swallowing difficulties, cardiac and respiratory disease, and the potential side-effects of medication.

It is important that parents and carers are given preventive guidance soon after diagnosis. Aggressive preventive therapies are essential, with oral hygiene aids provided when the need arises, as well as early access to regular dental attendance.

10.10 Myasthenia gravis

The name, 'serious muscle weakness', is an accurate description of this disease, which is due to a defect in the neurotransmission mechanism. Weakness is at its worst following exercise and seriously affects muscles of the face, tongue, neck, hands and feet. Generalised muscle weakness and fatigue may affect mobility, speech, eating and swallowing.

Typically, the lower jaw drops due to muscle weakness. Eating becomes an effort and dietary changes to facilitate mastication may result in an increased intake of soft or cariogenic food with an increase in contact time with teeth. Oral self-care may be tiring and difficult. Dental care when necessary is planned to coincide with periods when the individual suffers least fatigue, and general anaesthetics are avoided.

Symptoms are relieved with anticholinesterase, a drug which increases salivation. Atropine, which reduces salivary secretions, is sometimes prescribed, to enable the patient to cope with the high dosage of anticholinesterases. Steroids also provide relief, but their oral side-effects must be considered (Chapter 8).

10.11 Motor neurone disease

There are three types of this progressively disabling condition. Symptoms depend upon the site of the affected motor neurones. It is the physical aspects of weakness or paralysis in motor neurone disease which are the main factors in oral health. Weakness of head and neck muscles poses a risk to the airway, creates eating and swallowing difficulties, and causes real problems for oral care. Lubrication of the oral tissues is essential to maintain comfort. If the airway is compromised, techniques described for the dependent or dysphagic patient should be applied (Chapter 16).

10.12 Multiple sclerosis

Multiple sclerosis is a common neurological disorder caused by degeneration of the myelin sheath. It is extremely variable in the way it affects the sufferer, and is characterised by periods of remission and relapse. Physical symptoms include weakness, paralysis, tremors, loss of muscular co-ordination, and speech and swallowing difficulties. These symptoms limit oral self-care and access to services. Although there are no specific oral or dental problems, facial and oral hypersensitivity and anaesthesia may occur.

Sufferers have a higher incidence of trigeminal neuralgia, an acutely painful condition affecting areas of the face and mouth supplied by the trigeminal nerve. Relief may be provided by carbamazepine or phenytoin (*Colour Plate* 17), both of which have oral side-effects (Chapter 8).

Some relief and remission of neurological symptoms is provided by corticosteroids, which have oral side-effects. Drugs for the control of urinary incontinence may cause dry mouth. Preventive oral care is a priority.

10.13 Guillain-Barré syndrome

This is an acquired neuropathy which affects any age and is thought to be caused by a virus. In the acute phase, the patient may suffer from bilateral facial palsy and dysphagia, with variable motor and sensory loss in the limbs. Some 10–30% may have a range of residual disabilities[6]. Individual assessment at intervals during illness and in recovery ensures that the most appropriate oral care is provided. Chapter 16 provides guidance on oral care in dysphagia.

10.14 Stroke (cerebrovascular accident)

Stroke is a common cause of disability, especially in older people. Symptoms vary depending upon the area of the brain destroyed by haemorrhage. They may include weakness, loss of balance, paralysis, and speech and swallowing difficulties. With hemiplegia, personal care may be affected. Rehabilitation may involve the development of new skills with the non-dominant hand. If comprehension or communication is affected, this delays and interferes with rehabilitation.

One-sided facial paralysis mainly affects the lower part of the face; oral hygiene may deteriorate on the affected side due to muscle inactivity and the retention of food. Dentures appear to lose their fit due to lack of muscle control. If complete dentures are worn, sagging or drooping facial musculature can be supported and lifted by modifying the dentures on the affected side.

Swallowing difficulties increase contact between food and teeth. Dietary adjustment to maintain the nutritional status and assist with swallowing may increase the risk of dental caries. Patients receiving parenteral nutrition are still at risk of oral disease; calculus formation is significantly more rapid in tube-fed subjects compared with the non-tube-fed[7], indicating a significant oral care need. Some evidence suggests that fitting a palatal-training device improves the swallow reflex[8], although recovery and improvement may be spontaneous.

Physical Disability and Sensory Impairment

In the stroke patient, predisposing factors such as diabetes may affect oral health. Treatment for thrombotic or embolic causes with anticoagulants affects the management of dental care, as the anticoagulant dosage may need to be adjusted before dental extractions and some types of dental treatment. In the older person, the oral effects of multiple medication must be considered.

Interdisciplinary assessment should be carried out as early as possible to ensure that oral factors are included in the programme of rehabilitation. Minor adjustments to dentures to improve their stability or compensate for paralysis are relatively simple, and can make a significant contribution to the patient's condition. An oral care programme which takes account of the assessed and changing risk factors, in particular parenteral feeding, should be implemented at the outset[9].

10.15 Bell's palsy

Bell's palsy is the term for paralysis of the facial muscles caused by inflammation in the stylomastoid canal, although paralysis may be produced by other serious diseases, or following trauma or surgery. In Bell's palsy, paralysis develops quite rapidly and is generally preceded by pain in the area. It is usually unilateral and may also cause loss of taste. The prognosis for complete recovery is good, although some individuals have permanent residual paralysis.

Oral factors include drooling due to lack of muscular control on the affected side; this may be reduced by fitting an intra-oral appliance to lift the corner of the mouth or by modifying dentures, both of which are psychologically beneficial. Speech and swallowing may be affected. Food retained on the affected side is in increased contact with teeth, thus increasing the risk of caries and periodontal disease. A short course of steroids provides relief from the symptoms, and therefore the potential for oral side-effects should be limited.

10.16 Parkinson's disease

Parkinson's disease occurs most commonly in older people and is caused by degenerative changes in the basal ganglia leading to a shortage of the neurotransmitter, dopamine. Causative factors include cerebrovascular disease, head injury and viral infection, although parkinsonian-type symptoms may be secondary to psychiatric drugs, namely phenothiazines and butyrophenones (Chapters 8 and 12).

Features include tremor, which mainly affects arms and hands, rigidity of the limbs, and abnormal posture. Abnormal slowness in movement (akinesia) leads to immobility, and rigidity restricts activity, particularly the activities of daily living. Excessive salivation and drooling are due to delay and difficulty in swallowing rather than to an increase in the volume of saliva. Oral care may be obstructed by tremor or rigidity.

Treatment is mainly with anticholinergic drugs, such as orphenadrine and benzhexol, but levodopa in combination with other drugs is also effective. The side-effects of anticholinergics (*Table 10.2*) include dry mouth, which may help to reduce the problem of drooling but increases the potential for oral disease. Facial dyskinesia, involuntary movements of the facial muscles, such as pursing of the lips and 'flycatcher tongue', are distressing side-effects of levodopa and bromocriptine and may interfere with oral and dental care. The clinical aspects of denture construction can be particularly difficult.

10.17 Cleft lip and palate

Cleft lip and palate constitute one of the commonest forms of congenital malformation, which not only may be orally disabling but may also have consequences for speech, communication and learning, as well the psychological consequences of potential facial disfigurement and social acceptance. Cleft lip is more common in males, while cleft palate is commoner in females.

Although most cases are of genetic origin, other factors include nutritional deficiencies in pregnancy. It is reported that thalidomide, a known teratogenic drug, was associated with clefts, and an increased incidence of clefts may be associated with steroids.[10] They may also be associated with other congenital conditions, notably Down's syndrome, and other much rarer conditions, many of which are associated with a learning disability. Hearing impairment may also be a feature which complicates the development of speech, interferes with social development and delays learning.

Table 10.2 Oral side-effects of drugs used in Parkinson's disease.

Drug	*Oral side-effects*
Levodopa	Disturbances of taste (metallic)
	Abnormal facial movements
Bromocriptine	Dry mouth
	Abnormal facial movements
Amantadine hydrochloride	Dry mouth
Orphenadrine hydrochloride	Dry mouth
Benzhexol hydrochloride	Dry mouth
Benztropine mesylate	Dry mouth
Procyclidine	Dry mouth

Physical Disability and Sensory Impairment

The degree of involvement depends upon the structures affected. Clefts may involve just soft tissue or both soft and hard tissues and may be unilateral or bilateral. The more complex the defect, the greater the potential for disability. Facial deformities are the most obvious visible sign, while feeding difficulties may pose major problems, particularly in early childhood if the palate is affected. Obturators, oral appliances which cover the palatal defect, may be necessary for feeding and to assist with normal speech development.

Surgical repair of cleft lips is carried out at an early age, usually around three months, while palate repairs are generally completed by about 15 months, before the development of speech. Complex repairs may require multiple operations at various developmental stages; these may be complicated by other abnormalities. Susceptibility to upper respiratory tract infections may require frequent medication; the effect of sugar in medicines and the potential for dental caries has been highlighted in Chapters 3 and 8. Missing and malaligned teeth lead to problems with occlusion. Orthodontic treatment to correct these abnormalities may be complicated by post-operative scar tissue.

Cleft lip and palate pose a major risk of oral disability (*Colour Plate* **16**). Interdisciplinary assessment and treatment planning involving the paediatrician, maxillofacial team, speech therapists and others involved in primary care are usually initiated very soon after birth. Preventive programmes to include fluoride supplements in areas without water fluoridation, dietary advice and the development of good oral hygiene techniques, are vital, and should be implemented from birth.[11] All professionals involved in the care and treatment of clefts must be aware of the need and availability of lifetime preventive advice. The Cleft Lip and Palate Association (CLAPA)[12], a voluntary organisation of parents and professionals, has been set up to provide information, advice and support for people with clefts and their families.

10.18 Cerebral palsy

Cerebral palsy is one of the major causes of physical disability from birth. It has been included in this section, although approximately 50% have some other impairment or disability. These include visual, hearing and speech impairment, epilepsy, and learning disabilities (Chapter 11).

Restrictions imposed by physical disability limit access to dental care and to the management of oral care, while sensory and communication impairment have an impact on learning. Individual assessment is essential to establish whether delayed or slow learning is due to physical disability, mental disability or sensory impairment, or any combination of these factors.

The level and type of disability depends upon the area and degree of brain damage. Cerebral palsy results in a wide range of disability, from unnoticeable mild physical disability involving one limb (monoplegia), through to quadriplegia (all limbs). Movement may be affected and may be spastic, athetoid or ataxic.

Oral and dental disease in cerebral palsy

Children with a physical disability have been demonstrated to have higher levels of periodontal disease.[13,14] Other studies found no difference between the oral hygiene of children with cerebral palsy and their non-disabled siblings.[15] Although caries levels in cerebral palsy are similar to the 'normal' population, there is evidence that the average number of decayed, missing and filled teeth is higher in children with physical disability.[15]

Oral factors

Oral developmental abnormalities may affect oral health. Malocclusion caused by irregular teeth or an overcrowded mouth is common. Delayed eruption of the teeth contributes to malocclusion. Irregularities due to overcrowding interfere with effective plaque removal. Dietary changes to compensate for reduced masticatory ability may further increase the risk of caries.

Persistent grinding of the teeth (bruxism) causes the occlusal (biting) surfaces to wear flat (attrition) (*Colour Plate* 12). In some cases, this involuntary habit may wear the teeth down to the level of the gum. Flat biting surfaces are easy to clean and less prone to caries at the expense of the body of the tooth. Grinding teeth (bruxism) and involuntary muscle activity may put extra stress on the structures supporting the teeth predisposing to periodontal disease.

Oral reflexes may be impaired. These include the gag, cough, bite and swallowing reflexes and, when affected, feeding is difficult (Chapter 16). Impaired gag or cough reflexes place the individual at greater risk of aspiration when eating, while the bite reflex may persist beyond the normal age and interfere with feeding. Impaired reflexes may also pose restrictions on oral hygiene and dental treatment. A diet consisting of minced or soft foods, to help with swallowing, is more harmful to the teeth than whole or fibrous foods.

Dislocation of the jaw is relatively common. Chewing itself has a cleansing action in stimulating salivary flow. Difficulties or delay in swallowing increase contact times between food and teeth. People with cerebral palsy suffer acid regurgitation, and are therefore potentially more prone to acid erosion of enamel surfaces.

Poor co-ordination or manual disability may affect the individual's ability to care for their own mouth so the responsibility for maintaining oral hygiene will rest with a carer. Involuntary movements and impaired reflexes may mean that oral care is difficult to manage. Dental treatment may be difficult for both the patient and the dentist, so that treatment under general anaesthesia may be required.

Physical Disability and Sensory Impairment

Certain anticonvulsant drugs, which produce enlargement of the gingival margins (hyperplasia) (*Colour Plate* **17**), are described in Chapters 8 and 11. Dry mouth is a side-effect of antispasmodic medication and increases the risk to oral health. Oral factors are summarised in *Table 10.3*. Efficient and consistent plaque control can largely prevent side-effects. Chlorhexidine gluconate spray provides chemical plaque control when oral hygiene may be difficult.

Table 10.3 Oral aspects in cerebral palsy

• Malocclusion	• Acid regurgitation
• Bruxism	• Gag reflex
• Overcrowding	• Dietary factors
• Attrition	• Cough reflex
• Swallowing reflex	• Jaw dislocation
• Periodontal disease	• Anticonvulsant medication
• Chewing reflex	• Antispasmodic medication

Summary

A systematic pattern of preventive oral care should be established from birth to reduce the risk of caries and periodontal disease and the need for active dental treatment. The advice of a dentist or hygienist will be needed to identify the most appropriate care regime and preventive techniques. These should be reviewed at frequent intervals and modified accordingly. The dental team may also be involved in the construction of mouth-held appliances which assist with independence. Healthy teeth are a definite advantage in constructing a stable and useful mouthpiece (Chapter 9).

10.19 Spina bifida and hydrocephalus

Spina bifida and hydrocephalus may occur together or independently and are therefore covered together in this section.

Spina bifida

Spina bifida is a congenital defect caused by incomplete development of the spinal neural tube. In its simplest form, spina bifida occult, it is detected radiographically in approximately 50% of normal children and does not cause any physical or neurological abnormality. Spina bifida cystica, which is a major cause of paraplegia in children, occurs in two different forms, meningocele and myelomeningocele.

In meningocele, the meninges and cerebrospinal fluid protrude through a bony defect in the spinal column, forming a sac protruding from the vertebral column. It rarely produces neurological disability, although some 20% of those affected suffer from hydrocephalus. Defects are surgically corrected.

Myelomeningocele is the commonest type and is a serious defect where the spinal cord protrudes into the sac. It can occur at any point on the spine, although it is found mainly in the lumbar region. Paraplegia, with flaccid paralysis and loss of reflexes, loss of sensation and poor circulation, may occur as a result of damage to the spinal cord. Congenital hip dislocation is also common and hydrocephalus, epilepsy and learning disabilities are other complications.

Hydrocephalus

Hydrocephalus is caused by obstruction to the circulation of cerebrospinal fluid. It may be secondary to congenital conditions, infections, haemorrhage or tumours and cause brain damage due to pressure or atrophy. Unless treated, hydrocephalus leads to enlargement of the skull, brain damage, or death. Epilepsy, visual impairment, spasticity, and learning disabilities or dementia may present as complications. The insertion of a one-way valve which diverts cerebrospinal fluid away from the area releases pressure and has dramatically improved the prognosis. Valves may become dislodged or blocked and are regularly monitored.

There are no specific oral or dental features associated with spina bifida and hydrocephalus; however, paraplegia and the complications described may affect access to services, personal care and learning skills. Medication must be considered. The presence of a valve does pose problems for dental management; antibiotic cover is required for some forms of dental treatment to prevent potential infection of the valve which may lead to bacterial endocarditis (Chapter 13).

10.20 Spinal injuries and trauma

In modern industrial society, damage to the spinal cord is most commonly caused by traumatic injuries, mainly road traffic accidents or sports injuries. Rarely, it may be due to infections, haemorrhage, transverse myelitis, tumours or follow spinal surgery. Spinal cord injury is more prevalent in the under-40s, with young males affected more than young females. It can lead to severe disability in a previously fit person.

The sudden onset and severity of disability can understandably lead to a severe emotional reaction which influences the individual's ability to adjust to the dramatic changes in life-style, choice and dependence for personal needs.

The site and the severity of the lesion governs the type of disability. Cervical lesions are more seriously disabling, with a gradual potential

Physical Disability and Sensory Impairment

for increased function the lower the injury. The effect is paralysis and loss of sensation in the areas receiving their nervous supply at, or below, the injured area. Paraplegia refers to injury below the cervical vertebrae resulting in paralysis of the lower limbs, and tetraplegia (quadriplegia) to injury in the cervical region resulting in paralysis of all limbs and the trunk to varying degrees. With incomplete transection of the spinal cord, limited function and sensation may return. With lower cervical injury some arm movements may be possible, although hands may be weak, lacking power, and dexterity (*Table 10.4*).

Apart from functional and sensory disabilities, spasticity, pain, tremors and urinary infections are among the symptoms which may require treatment with medication. Antibiotics, muscle relaxants and analgesics should be checked for their potential for oral side-effects.

Tetraplegics with high cervical lesions and intercostal paralysis may require a respirator or tracheostomy and will be totally dependent for personal care. The cough and gag reflexes may be affected. It is important to ensure that appropriate oral care is implemented at the outset. In the early stages of rehabilitation, oral hygiene techniques may be limited to those described in Chapter 16. With lower cervical injuries, adaptive equipment may be required to stabilise the wrist, support the arm and to facilitate grasping (Chapter 9).

Self-caring skills must be individually assessed and encouraged by a team approach and the appropriate aids provided (Chapter 9). The dental team may be involved in restoring any damaged teeth, developing oral care plans, providing preventive advice and treatment, selecting aids to facilitate oral self-care, and in the construction of mouth appliances to increase independence.

Table 10.4 Potential consequences of complete spinal cord damage.

Injury level	*Motor loss*	*Sensory loss*
C1 to C4 Quadriplegia	Paralysis of diaphragm, intercostal muscles with flaccid total paralysis below the neck	From the neck downwards
C5 to C8 Paraplegia	Paralysis of intercostal muscles, below shoulders and upper arms	Arms, hands, chest, abdomen and lower limbs
T1 to T6 Paraplegia	Paralysis below the mid chest	Below the mid chest
T7 to T12 Paraplegia	Paralysis below waist	Below waist
T12 to L1	Paralysis in most leg muscles and in pelvis	Lower abdomen and legs

10.21 Head injury

Although head injuries affect relatively few of the population of the UK, the numbers increase by approximately 2,000 a year. Progress in resuscitation techniques and neuro-surgical management have increased survival rates. Headway[16] reports that the average general medical practitioner probably has no more than two severely head-injured patients registered with the practice, thus knowledge of the effects is limited. However, the head-injured and their families experience considerable stress and stigma due to personality changes – hidden disabilities which are not easily recognised.

Trauma to the head is largely due to road traffic accidents. Resultant disabilities do not fit easily into the major disability categories. Since physical disability may be a feature, and since they have received little recognition as a group, head-injured patients are included in this section. Residual disability depends upon the nature and severity of the head injury, speed and level of expertise in management and the individual's previous personality, ability and skills. Apart from any visible physical disability, various problems may be encountered. These are listed in *Table 10.5*, along with symptoms that may occur.

Table 10.5 Head-injured patients: possible problems and symptoms.

Problems:	Personality changes
	Depression
	Memory loss and poor recall
	Frustration
	Poor concentration and motivation
	Mood changes
	Comprehension
	Inhibition
	Tiredness and lethargy
Symptoms:	Epilepsy (Chapters 11, 12)
	Changes in sexual drive
	Difficulty using hands and limbs
	Dizziness
	Speech difficulties
	Sensory deprivation
	Headaches
	Weakness or hemiplegia

In functional terms, skills which enable the individual to perform the activities of daily living may be lost. Self-care may be replaced by dependence, even though there is no visible reason for this, and the image created in the lay person's mind is of a learning disability. Coping with these personality changes and changed behaviour creates stressful pres-

Physical Disability and Sensory Impairment

sures on the head-injured person, his or her family and friends.

In terms of oral health, severe physical disability will create dependence for oral care (Chapter 16). Visual neglect, when the individual is cognitively unaware of one half of the visual field or body, may affect the mouth. Transference of skills from the dominant hand may affect manual skills. Visual agnosia is demonstrated by the inability to recognise common objects such as a toothbrush or toothpaste. Memory loss may interfere with previously acquired skills, while cognitive deficit may lead to difficulty with the sequence of activities in simple tasks such as toothbrushing. These are features which may affect any individual suffering from organic brain damage.

The management of rehabilitation involves inter-disciplinary assessment, including rehabilitation medicine, neuropsychology, speech therapy, physiotherapy, occupational therapy and, of course, the family, to develop individual programmes for independence. The dental team needs to be involved in programmes which relate to oral care skills; regular domiciliary visits from a dental hygienist may be necessary to support the family or carers in maintaining oral health. The primary care team should ensure that regular dental care is available.

10.22 Epilepsy

Approximately 1% of the population suffer from epilepsy. It is the commonest neurological disorder, after migraine, and causes disturbances of consciousness of motor or sensory function. It is commoner in children and people with learning disabilities, but it may present as a symptom of organic brain disease or as a consequence of head injury, substance abuse, or metabolic disorders.[17]

There may also be psychiatric problems due to social stigma, with consequent repercussions upon the individual's personal and social integration and personality.[18] The oral side-effects of antipsychotic medication need to be considered, in addition to the side-effects of anticonvulsive therapy and oral trauma during seizures.

Accidental injury to the teeth may occur during convulsions and there is a greater incidence of fractured or damaged teeth (*Colour Plate* **17**). Sometimes fragments of teeth and roots which are buried in the jaw bone or soft tissues lay dormant for long periods. They can be identified by X-ray and may be the cause of acute pain and infection.

Medication, notably phenytoin, used to control convulsions, causes enlargement and sometimes tenderness of the gums around the teeth (*Colour Plate* **17**). In its most severe form, the teeth may become submerged beneath the gingival overgrowth. Alternative drugs are available; however, side-effects are always secondary to the importance of controlling convulsions. Enlargement of the gums (gingival hyperplasia) associated with phenytoin can be largely prevented by good plaque control. One oral side-effect of carbamazepine, prescribed as an anticonvulsant, is to reduce saliva; reduced salivary flow increases the risk of caries and periodontal disease.

Dentures are generally not advised for people who suffer from severe epilepsy because of the risk of inhaling parts of a broken denture, so it is particularly important whenever possible to avoid tooth loss and the need for dentures. In many cases the dentist will not construct dentures without first seeking the advice of the neurologist. If dentures are made, they may be constructed from a radio-opaque plastic, which is unfortunately weaker than normal denture plastic. Metal dentures are a possible alternative, but each case is assessed individually. Oral factors are summarised in *Table 10.6*.

Table 10.6 Epilepsy: oral factors.

Fracture
Buried roots
Denture problems
Gingival hyperplasia
Anticonvulsant medication

10.23 Sensory impairment

Visual and hearing impairments are often overlooked in disability issues, and yet sensory impairments are extremely common. Although sensory impairment does not cause a physical disability, possible barriers to oral health include communication, information, access, services and professional attitudes.

Visual impairment

Whereas visual defects are commonly genetic, some are associated with other conditions which may lead to visual impairment, e.g diabetes mellitus or viral infections. Oral hygiene may be inadequate in individuals with no visual feedback on the standard of their oral hygiene. Gingivitis increases if oral hygiene is poor, while oral and facial trauma may be more frequent due to falls and accidental injury. Studies have demonstrated that oral hygiene is significantly worse in a blind population than in an equivalent sighted population.[19,20]

Teaching oral hygiene skills must take into account the lack of visual feedback and maximise the use of tactile skills.[21] To compensate for this, a Touch Tooth Kit has been developed to teach oral hygiene skills to children with severe visual impairment.[22]

Physical Disability and Sensory Impairment

Hearing impairment

There are no specific oral and dental problems associated with hearing impairment, except in rare cases, when it is associated with congenital conditions such as Treacher Collins or rubella syndrome, learning disabilities or cardiac disease.

In rubella syndrome, enamel defects may occur and bruxism (persistent grinding) may be a feature. Sensitive and skilled communication may be necessary to teach oral hygiene and the correct measures for maintaining oral health.

10.24 Summary

This chapter summarises the commonest disabling conditions which may affect mobility and manual dexterity. Many rarer conditions to which the same principles can be applied have not been covered. The chapter summarises specific oral problems which pose an increased risk of oral disease together with the oral side-effects of treatment.

With increased dependence, oral care skills may be lost. Oral health may deteriorate, reducing the potential quality of life and increasing the possibility of crisis management for the relief of pain. To avoid this and reduce the burden on carers, referral and advice should be provided whenever possible, soon after diagnosis. Health care professionals are in a prime position to initiate this process and provide informed advice and support.

10.25 References

1. Martin, J., Meltzer, H. and Elliot, D. (1988). *The Prevalence of Disability Among Adults: Report 1*. London, HMSO.
2. Edwards, F.C. and Warren, M.D. (1990). *Health Services for Adults with Physical Disabilities. A Survey of District Health Authorities 1988/89*. London, The Royal College of Physicians of London.
3. Phillips, P.L. and Brunner, A. (1990). 'But sometimes you do say Help!'. Report on a survey of people with long-term health problems or physical disabilities in NE Essex between June and November 1990. Colchester, North East Essex Health Authority.
4. Khaligh, N. and Wood, P.N.H. (1986). *Arthritis and Rheumatism in the Eighties*. London, Arthritis Care, p. 5.
5. World Health Organisation Chronicle. (1979).
6. Scully, C. and Cawson, R.A. (1987). *Medical Problems in Dentistry*. 2nd ed., Bristol, Wright, p. 315.

7. Dicks, J.L. and Banning, J. (1991). Evaluation of calculus accumulation in tube-fed mentally handicapped patients: the effects of oral hygiene status. *Spec. Care in Dent.*, **11**(3), 104–106.
8. Oliver, R.G. (1987). Theoretical aspects and clinical experience with the palatal training appliance for saliva control in persons with cerebral palsy. *Spec. Care in Dent.*, Nov.–Dec., 271–274.
9. Raha, S, Finucane, P. and Duncan, D. (1991). Percutaneous endoscopic gastrostomy. *Br. J. Hosp. Medicine*, **46**(1), 53–54.
10. Scully, C. and Cawson, R.A. (1987). *Medical Problems in Dentistry.* 2nd ed. Bristol, Wright, p. 419.
11. Thom, A.R. (1990). Modern management of the cleft lip and palate patient. *Dental Update*, Dec., 402–408.
12. Cleft Lip and Palate Association, The National Secretary, 1 Eastwood Gardens, Kenton, Newcastle upon Tyne, NE3 3DQ.
13. Lyons, D. (1960). The dental health of a group of handicapped adolescent children. *J. Clin. Periodontol.*, **31**, 52.
14. Miller, J.B. and Taylor, P.P. (1970). A survey of the oral health of a group of orthopaedically handicapped children. *J. Dent. Child.*, **37**, 331.
15. Fishman, S.T., Young, W.O., Haley, J.B. *et al.* (1967). The status of oral health in cerebral palsied children and their siblings. *J. Dent. Child.*, **34**, 219.
16. Headway, National Head Injuries Association Ltd., 7 King Edward Court, Nottingham, NG1 1EW.
17. Stafford-Clark, D., Bridges, P. and Black, D. (1990). *Psychiatry for Students.* 7th ed. London, Unwin Hyman, p. 111–113.
18. Hughes, A.M. *et al.* (1989). Psychiatric disorders in a dental clinic. *Br. Dent. J.*, **166**, 16–19.
19. Anaise, J.Z. (1976). Periodontal disease and oral hygiene in a group of blind and sighted teenagers in Israel (14–17 years of age). *J. Dent Child.*, **7**, 353–356.
20. Greeley, C.B., Goldstein, P.A. and Forrester, D.J. (1976). Oral manifestations in a group of blind students. *J. Dent. Child.*, **43**, 39–42.
21. O'Donnell, D. and Crosswaite, M.A. (1991). Dental health education for the visually impaired child. *Dental Health*, **30**(1), 8–9.
22. Cleary, J.L and Valentine, A.D. (1988). The 'Touch Tooth' Kit. *Dental Practice*, **26**(1), 1–3.

11 People with Learning Disabilities

11.1 Introduction
11.2 Barriers to dental care
11.3 Oral and dental health
11.4 Risk factors
11.5 Down's syndrome
11.6 Cerebral palsy
11.7 Epilepsy
11.8 Autism
11.9 Oral self-mutilation
11.10 Medicines and drugs
11.11 Preventive measures
11.12 Summary
11.13 Pamphlets
11.14 References

11.1 Introduction

This chapter discusses the specific oral and dental problems which may be experienced by people with 'learning disabilities'. The term 'mental handicap' is widely used and understood by professionals, carers, and the public generally. However, 'people with learning disabilities' is the current term for this group of people, although the debate over terminology is continuing.

'Learning disabilities' conforms with the use of non-stigmatising language, and is the preferred term of articulate members of this group. People who are profoundly or multiply handicapped are generally assumed to have severe learning disabilities.

Apart from a few very rare conditions, this group has the same oral and dental problems as the rest of the population. They suffer from dental caries (decay) and periodontal (gum) disease leading to tooth loss. Daily oral care to reduce plaque and dietary control of sugars should therefore be a matter of routine. However, this group has poorer oral health than the general population, a fact which is confirmed by studies of various populations with a learning disability.

In Chapter 2, it was clearly shown that effective oral care requires knowledge, skill and motivation. Many so-called self-caring adults, who should be able to manage their own oral care, have already lost their natural teeth. If

Holistic Oral Care

learning is restricted or impaired, or the individual is not motivated to carry out effective oral care, an increased risk of oral disease is inevitable.

For some, the techniques for maintaining oral health will be more difficult to learn, and regular supervision may be required, while supervision and assistance will be essential for other individuals. The profoundly or multiply handicapped are likely to be completely dependent with regard to the maintenance of oral health and therefore reliant upon the knowledge and skills of their carers.

Caring for the mouth is one aspect of personal care. Plaque must be removed efficiently for oral hygiene to be effective, and most people need individual advice if oral care is to be effective.

Without good oral hygiene and prevention, pain is an almost inevitable consequence. In some cases, because of neglect or the individual's inability to co-operate, the only way of relieving pain is tooth extraction under general anaesthesia. The loss of natural teeth may add an extra burden to an individual who may already be disadvantaged, and may result in a dental handicap. The use of dentures to compensate for tooth loss requires learning new skills to control and use dentures. If a person cannot wear dentures, this adds a further burden and disadvantage and may lead to an oral and/or social handicap.

Regardless of the type of learning disability, the principles of plaque control and reduction of dietary sugars are universal. Carers have an important role in helping their children/wards or patients/clients to maintain their health and independence. The role of carers, whether informal or professional, is to teach, encourage, assist and, to a very large extent, to provide oral care. They will also need to ensure that preventive measures are implemented regularly, to encourage a healthy diet, and to ensure regular contact with the dental services.

11.2 Barriers to dental care

Traditional barriers to dental care exist in this group, such as:

- Oral health may have a low priority in the family context of coping with disability.
- Dental care may be restricted by attitudes and access.
- Treatment may be more difficult to provide because of fear and anxiety, lack of understanding, inability to co-operate or challenging behaviour.
- Involuntary movements may restrict oral care or dental treatment.
- Difficulties with communication complicate the situation.

It may help to overcome these barriers if a familiar relationship has been established by regular contact with the dental team from the individual's birth or early childhood. For those with challenging behaviour or more profound handicaps, it may be necessary to use specialist dental services which are usually available from both the Community and Hospital Dental Services.

11.3 Oral and dental health

It is reported that people with learning disabilities have poorer oral health than the so-called 'normal' population. Surveys of the oral health and treatment needs of this group are not extensive, but generally confirm inequalities in oral health. Most British studies have been carried out in special schools, adult training centres and institutions. Although studies differ in methodology, they show that these groups have higher levels of tooth loss and periodontal (gum) disease and poorer oral hygiene. Levels of dental caries (decay) are generally similar to comparable populations, although there is evidence that more decayed teeth remain untreated.

Evidence of dental neglect is provided by the higher numbers of teeth lost by extraction found in this group. This suggests that dental treatment has been less available or less accessible. Delays in receiving treatment may lead to a higher proportion of extractions. The evidence seems to confirm the historic treatment pattern of extractions rather than fillings for people with learning disabilities.

Plaque and periodontal disease

Studies, confirming the high levels of periodontal disease, high levels of plaque and low standards of oral hygiene which are reported, refer mainly to the child population.[1,2] Plaque levels are highest in institutionalised populations, and increase with age, while periodontal conditions are worst in people with severe learning disabilities.

Certain conditions associated with a learning disability pose an increased risk of periodontal disease. The side-effects of long-term medication increase oral health risks. The implications of specific conditions and medication are discussed in later sections. Preventive measures, in addition to plaque control, must therefore have a very high priority in these groups. Chemical plaque control may be essential to compensate for difficulties in maintaining oral health.

Dental decay

Generally, the number of decayed teeth in this group differs very little from that of 'normal' groups. However, it is found that decay is more extensive and more teeth are lost due to untreated decay.[1] Institutionalised people have less dental caries than those living in the community, and it is suggested that restricted access to cariogenic food and snacking are a contributory factor. A closer look reveals the inequalities in dental caries in this group.

A number of studies have found that institutionalised children experience less dental caries than 'handicapped' or 'normal' children living in the community. However, the institutionalised groups have higher numbers of missing teeth.[3] In several other studies, fewer fillings had been given and there were a higher proportion of untreated decayed teeth in children with learning disabilities as compared with normal children[3].

In contrast, a Swedish study has demonstrated that improved resources benefited children with severe learning disabilities so that there was no neglected need for treatment.[4]

Although, in 1976, the Court Report highlighted the higher levels of dental disease in handicapped children and made recommendations for improvements in dental health[5], the situation has not significantly improved since then. A more recent review of the literature confirms the generally continuing levels of untreated caries present in handicapped children.[6]

Needs of this sector

Poor oral hygiene, poor plaque control and more periodontal disease are consistently reported in studies of people with learning disabilities as compared with 'normal' populations. Although levels of dental caries are generally comparable with 'normal' populations, more teeth are lost through extraction. There is a higher unmet need for dental treatment in this group. The dental profession is concerned to reduce these inequalities and promote the oral health of this group. These are factors which must be considered in the process of normalisation and the development of community care.

11.4 Risk factors

A number of factors place individuals in this group at greater risk of developing oral disease. Oral and dental health may be complicated by medical or behavioural factors and their treatment. Soft diets compensating for the inability to chew and abnormal muscle activity both contribute to the higher rate of periodontal disease.

The commonest conditions are discussed, although any of the factors described might apply to the rarer syndromes and other causes of learning disability and profound mental handicap.

11.5 Down's syndrome

Down's syndrome is caused by a chromosomal abnormality, and is the commonest clinically classifiable condition associated with a learning disability.[7] The development of foetal tests to identify chromosomal abnormalities and the possibility of termination are likely to reduce the number of those born with Down's syndrome. Apart from characteristic physical features, there are both physical and medical aspects which affect oral health and dental management. A description of the condition is necessary to understand the risks to oral health and the implications for dental treatment. People with Down's syndrome tend to have a physically short stature with fairly recognisable facial characteristics. Abnormal development of the jaws and teeth are also a feature. Other physiological abnormalities will be described.

Oral and dental disease

There is an increased susceptibility to periodontal disease compared with other groups with learning disabilities[3], which is widely recognised as the most important dental disorder in Down's syndrome. Children with Down's syndrome have similar plaque levels to other age-related groups, but higher levels of periodontal disease.[3]

Lower levels of periodontal disease are reported among those living at home than among those institutionalised.[8] This suggests that care and motivation in toothbrushing and plaque control, dietary and other environmental factors, may counteract the tendency towards poor periodontal health. There may be other factors, as yet unresearched, which contribute to the high levels of periodontal disease.

Lower levels of caries are reported among children with Down's syndrome than in other children with learning disabilities[9]. However, fewer teeth were found to be present because of delayed eruption and congenitally missing teeth.

Oral factors

Abnormal jaw development is characterised by a small upper jaw (maxilla) and sometimes a larger and protruding lower jaw (mandible). There is an increased incidence of cleft lip and palate. Developmental abnormalities cause problems in the way in which teeth in both arches meet. Such abnormalities (malocclusions) may reduce the ability to chew efficiently; the cleansing action of chewing is thus lost. A soft diet may be recommended to compensate for reduced masticatory ability, but this has the potential for accumulation of food debris, thus increasing the risk of oral disease.

Lips, which may be thick, dry and fissured, often assume a lips-apart posture, exposing the underlying gingivae. This can cause localised dryness of the gums, predisposing to periodontal disease. An open-mouth posture due to mouth-breathing has a similar effect.

Other abnormalities include a large tongue with a tendency to a forward tongue thrust. This may affect the individual's or the carer's ability to carry out effective oral hygiene techniques, and poses problems for the management of dental treatment.

Tooth eruption is often delayed with the primary teeth starting to erupt as late as nine months and ending at about five years. Teeth may be abnormally shaped with short crowns and roots, and some teeth do not develop. The abnormal shape of teeth and the irregularities which occur are more likely to lead to the accumulation of food debris and plaque. Oral factors are summarised in *Table 11.1*.

Table 11.1 Down's syndrome: oral factors.

- Abnormal jaw relationships
- Cleft lip and palate
- Malocclusions
- Reduced masticatory ability
- Poor lip posture
- Mouth-breathing
- Large tongue
- Abnormal-shaped crowns
- Missing teeth
- Anticonvulsant medication

Physiological factors

About 50% of those born with Down's syndrome have some form of congenital heart disease, and cardiac abnormalities are the major cause of death in the first few years of life. Apart from the obvious effects of cardiac disease in reducing the quality of life, heart defects pose a risk for dental treatment.

When teeth are scaled or extracted, bacteria normally present in the mouth enter the bloodstream, creating a bacteraemia. In a healthy individual this does not pose a problem. However, in congenital heart disease, bacteria settle on the damaged areas, causing endocarditis (inflammation of the lining of the heart), a serious and potentially fatal condition.

Fortunately, bacterial endocarditis can be prevented by taking an antibiotic before and, in certain circumstances, after dental treatment (Chapter 13). Dental management is therefore affected and the need for an accurate medical history before dental treatment is given cannot be stressed too heavily.

Respiratory problems predispose to upper respiratory tract infections, and pulmonary hypertension and chronic obstructive airway disease occur more frequently. If cardiac or respiratory disease is a feature, dental treatment requiring a general anaesthetic should be carried out under hospital conditions.

Defects in the immune system are a feature of Down's syndrome, and increase the risk of skin, respiratory and gastric disease. It is thought that immunodeficiency may be a major contributory factor to the development of periodontal disease.

A higher incidence of hepatitis B carrier status is reported, particularly in institutions, and immunodeficiency is believed to lead to a poor antibody response to hepatitis B. The increased incidence of hepatitis B carrier status poses problems for dental management and cross-infection control. The incidence of acute leukaemia in Down's syndrome is ten times greater than in the general population. Oral signs of leukaemia include anaemia, gingivitis (inflammation of the gums), ulceration and oral infections (Chapter 15). Leukaemia may initially be diagnosed by a dentist, as the individual may present with oral symptoms.

Atlanto-axial (cervical) instability occurs in some individuals with Down's syndrome. Care must be taken in extending the neck to avoid dislocation. This has implications for managing oral care, dental treatment and providing a general anaesthetic (*Table 11.2*).

Table 11.2 Down's syndrome: medical aspects.

- Congenital heart disease
- Leukaemia
- Respiratory disease
- Atlanto-axial instability
- Immunodeficiency
- General anaesthetic risk
- Higher risk of hepatitis B
- Anticonvulsant medication

Learning skills

People with Down's syndrome show a wide range in intellectual capacities, from mild to severe learning disabilities. Integration into mainstream education and employment features highly in the programme of normalisation and social role valorisation. Many can, and will, fulfil a socio-economic role in society provided that attitudinal barriers are overcome.

Individual assessment of intellectual ability is necessary to teach appropriate oral hygiene skills. A carer may ultimately bear the responsibility for teaching, motivation or managing oral care. Hearing and visual defects may complicate learning. Hearing defects are common, and visual defects leading to cataracts occur in some 50% of sufferers by the age of 50. Problems with visual accommodation need to be considered when teaching oral hygiene skills which rely on visual feedback.

Both premature ageing and a higher incidence of Alzheimer's disease occur in those with Down's syndrome. Medical advances mean that more Down's syndrome individuals survive into middle age and later life. Depression in middle age and personality deterioration may signify the onset of dementia. Epilepsy is reported in approximately 50% of those who show early signs of general deterioration[9], and when treated with anticonvulsants, the oral side-effects may affect oral health (Chapter 8). With depression, premature ageing and dementia, the skills required for oral hygiene or associated with the wearing of new dentures may be difficult or impossible to learn (*Table 11.3*).

Table 11.3 Down's syndrome: behavioural aspects.

- Oral hygiene skills
- Motivation
- Co-operation
- Communication
- Visual accommodation
- Depression
- Premature ageing
- Alzheimer's disease

The complex physical and medical problems described in Down's syndrome and summarised in *Tables 11.1–11.3* identify this group of individuals as more at risk of oral disease. Periodontal disease is a significant problem, and good plaque control is therefore essential whether managed by the individual or carer. Chemical plaque control in the form of chlorhexidine mouthwash, gel or spray (Chapter 9) may be a necessary aid to plaque control.

Dental treatment poses additional risks if a general anaesthetic is required. A programme to establish preventive oral and dietary habits and regular dental attendance should be set up at an early age to maintain oral health and reduce the need for dental intervention.

11.6 Cerebral palsy

Cerebral palsy is discussed in detail in Chapter 10 on physical disability, although approximately 50% of those affected will also have some other impairment or disability. These include visual, hearing and speech impairment, epilepsy and learning disabilities. Individual assessment is essential to establish an appropriate oral care programme from birth.

11.7 Epilepsy

This neurological symptom has been discussed in Chapter 10. Behavioural problems associated with a learning disability may interfere with oral care and pose a greater risk to the individual's oral health. The oral side-effects of phenytoin are worse when plaque control is poor. This group needs special attention in controlling plaque and chemical plaque control may be essential if co-operation is limited. Chlorhexidine delivered by spray may be accepted or tolerated when toothbrushing is difficult or impossible.

11.8 Autism

This condition is characterised by a failure to develop interpersonal relationships, with delayed speech and communication and a fascination with inanimate objects. Many autistic individuals have a learning disability, although some are highly intelligent. The sense of behavioural isolation may impair learning. Epilepsy develops in approximately 30% of those affected.

Communication and comprehension may affect oral care and co-operation for care and treatment. Epilepsy and behavioural problems, such as head-banging, increase the risk of fractured teeth. The possible effects of medication should also be considered.

11.9 Oral self-mutilation

Self-inflicted injuries to the head and mouth may occur in emotionally disturbed individuals. In Lesch–Nyhan syndrome, a rare metabolic cause of learning disability, the individual compulsively chews the lips and tongue or may self-injure the face, head or hands. Self-mutilation may also occur in Gilles de la Tourette's syndrome. In Riley–Day syndrome, self-injury may be accidental due to congenital indifference to pain. In Pica syndrome, which is characterised by the ingestion of unnatural or inedible foods, trauma may be caused to the oral tissues.

One of the authors has extracted 16 primary teeth from a six-year-old child in order to prevent total destruction of the lips and tongue. Scar tissue in the lips resulted in serious facial disfigurement and created malocclusion in the secondary dentition which interfered with the child's ability to chew. A soft diet was necessary to provide adequate nutrition which increased the risk of dental caries. Orthodontic treatment was not practical due to the severity of the child's handicap. This might have been avoided if the agreed procedure for all new patients to be referred for oral assessment on admission had been used.

It is important to be aware of the potential risk of self-inflicted injury. Care must be taken to protect the individual from self-mutilation and to prevent accidental self-injury following dental treatment under local or general anaesthesia. A soft plastic splint which covers the biting surfaces may be required to prevent post-anaesthetic self-mutilation.[10]

11.10 Medicines and drugs

People suffering from chronic illness may require long-term medication, but due to problems in its administration, medicines with a high sugar concentration may be prescribed more often. The practice of administering medicines last thing at night, when the salivary flow is reduced, increases the risk of caries.

Apart from some of the drugs used to control epilepsy, which have already been mentioned, other drugs may cause oral side-effects such as xerostomia, ulceration and soreness. These may impair oral hygiene techniques, and the advice of a dentist should be obtained.

A dry mouth increases the risk of caries and periodontal disease. Good oral hygiene is essential, and sweetened sugary drinks should be avoided as a means of relieving a dry mouth. Water provides the safest and simplest relief (Chapters 2 and 8).

11.11 Preventive measures

Diagnosis at birth or an early age offers an opportunity to reinforce parental advice and guidance on the need for appropriate preventive measures, dietary control of sugars and regular dental attendance as a means of preventing dental health problems in adult life.[11]

The educational role of the primary care nurse in post-natal and pre-school contact with children is paramount in providing parents with the necessary information and support in establishing a preventive regime. Possible risk factors are summarised in *Table 11.4*.

Table 11.4 Risk factors.

Family value of oral health	Manual disability
Motivation	Inadequate oral care
Learning ability	Crisis orientation to care
Prolonged bottle feeding	Malocclusion (*Colour Plate* 15)
Special or inadequate diets	Overcrowding (*Colour Plate* 15)
Cariogenic foods as a reward	Poor muscular co-ordination
Sugar-based medicines	Anti-convulsant medication
Motor dysfunction	

The basis of preventive advice includes measures such as mechanical and chemical plaque control, dietary control of extrinsic sugars, fluoride toothpastes and supplements, and alternatives to sugar-based medicines. Early registration with a dentist to provide advice on individual problems and referral to a dental hygienist are essential; the Community Dental Service is at present the most appropriate primary dental care service for people with severe learning disabilities living in the community.

11.12 Summary

People with learning disabilities have poorer oral health and a greater unmet need for treatment. In the debate about normalisation and social role valorisation, it is important that, in increasing choice, this group is not denied access to improved oral health and, if necessary, appropriate specialist dental services. Carers, whether family, professional or voluntary, need to know the risks to oral health and about various preventive techniques, so that their charges' oral health and dignity can be maintained. In turn, this will help to increase their rightful social acceptance in society.

11.13 Pamphlets

The Handicapped Child Starts with Healthy Teeth. (Nieuwegein), Holland, Association for the Advancement of Dentistry for the Handicapped.
Healthy mouth, happy smile. For your child who may need special help. (London), General Dental Council, British Society of Dentistry for the Handicapped and British Paedodontic Society.
Scully, C. *Something to Bite On: Dental Care for Mentally Handicapped Children.* London, National Society for Mentally Handicapped Children.

11.14 References

1. Brown, J.P. and Schodel, D.R. (1976). A review of controlled surveys of dental disease in handicapped persons. *J. Dentistry for Children*, **43**, 313–320.
2. Tesini, D.A. (1981). An annotated review of the literature of dental caries and periodontal disease in mentally retarded individuals. *Special Care Dentist*, **1**, 75.
3. Hunter, B. (1987). *Dental Care for Handicapped Patients.* Bristol, Wright, pp. 6–13.
4. Forsberg, H., Quick-Nilsson, I. and Gustavson, K. (1985). Dental health and dental care in severely mentally retarded children. *Swedish Dent. Jour.*, **9**, 15.
5. Court, S.D.M. (1976). *Fit for the Future. Report of the Committee on Child Health.* Cmnd no. 6684. London, HMSO.
6. Nunn, J.H. (1987). The dental health of mentally and physically handicapped children: a review of the literature. *Community Dental Health*, **4**, 157–168.
7. Scully, C. and Cawson, R.A. (1987). *Medical Problems in Dentistry.* 2nd ed. Bristol, Wright, pp. 410–412.
8. Lott, I.T. and Lai, F. (1982). Dementia in Down's syndrome: observations from a neurology clinic. *Applied Research in Mental Retardation*, **3**, 233–239.
9. Cutress, T.W. (1971). Periodontal disease and oral hygiene in Trisomy 21. *Arch. Oral Biol.*, **16**, 1345.
10. Crespi, P.V. and Friedman, R.B. (1986). Prevention of post-anaesthetic oral self-mutilation. *Spec. Care in Dent.*, March–April, 68–69.
11. Miller, J. and Barmes, D.E. (1980). Oral health. In: Falkner, F. *Prevention in Childhood of Health Problems in Adult Life.* Geneva, World Health Organisation, pp. 107–119.

12 People Suffering From Mental Illness

12.1 Introduction
12.2 Oral health and disease
12.3 Barriers to oral health
12.4 Side-effects of medication
12.5 Neuroses
12.6 Psychoses
12.7 Psychosomatic disorders
12.8 Anorexia nervosa and bulimia
12.9 Alcohol and substance abuse
12.10 People with learning difficulties
12.11 Children and adolescents
12.12 Summary
12.13 References

12.1 Introduction

This chapter discusses the oral and dental problems associated with mental illness. Brief accounts of conditions are given to provide the reader with a reference point in relation to behaviour which may affect oral health.

Mental illness is a broad term for a number of diagnosed and undiagnosed psychological conditions of varying types and degrees which may contribute to emotional and social disability or even handicap. The borderline between mental health and mental illness is very fine and largely culturally defined.

Conditions consistent with a diagnosis of 'mental illness or distress' are estimated to affect 1 in 10 of the UK population annually, or about six million people.[1] Estimates are based upon diagnosis through contact with general medical services and are probably an underestimate of the true prevalence. The lifetime prevalence rate in the USA is approximately 25% of the population[2], with 6% affected by serious affective disorders.[3]

Mental illness is virtually confined to the adult population, with more women than men being affected and with most cases – approximately 4.5 million – occurring in those aged between 15 and 64 years, with a further 1.2 million in those over 65 years of age.[1] Although the prevalence of mental illness in children is very low, the possible effects on parenting must be considered if one or both parents suffer from mental illness.

People Suffering from Mental Illness

The prevalence of mental illness compares with cardiac and circulatory disorders as a major health problem in the UK. Diagnostic labels fall into three main categories: psychoses, neuroses and 'other forms', which are broadly behavioural and stress-related disorders.

Intrinsic causes, such as recognisable organic brain disease, affect relatively few individuals except in the older age groups, while some systemic diseases may also lead to psychiatric problems. In certain conditions, heredity may be a contributory factor, and in conditions such as Huntington's chorea it is a known factor. The incidence of Alzheimer's disease in people with Down's syndrome may be related to premature ageing and/or genetic factors.[4]

Behaviour associated with alcohol or substance abuse may have a psychiatric component. The effects of major trauma or severe life-threatening conditions may lead to a range of individual emotional reactions. Biochemical factors associated with endocrinal changes are suggested causes of post-natal or menopausal depression, although extrinsic factors cannot be excluded. Physical illness and biochemical deficiencies are also quoted as possible intrinsic factors.

Extrinsic factors, such as stress, family or social pressures and poor or inadequate housing, are contributory. Females are generally more often admitted to hospital for all mental illnesses, especially for depressive illness. Some disorders appear to have a higher incidence in certain racial groups, while the prevalence of schizophrenia appears to be higher in social classes IV and V, although the stigma attached to the condition and the subsequent downward drift may account for the reported class distribution.[5]

Pressure to achieve has led to an increased value attached to individual success, autonomy and self-reliance, with a concomitant devaluation of the non-achiever. Stress as a factor in both organic and mental illness is increasingly accepted as an aetiological factor. An isolated and relatively insignificant incident in the context of other factors may be the precipitating factor.

Historical patterns of custodial care in large psychiatric institutions are changing. The gradual closure of institutions and the provision of care at home or in sheltered and supported community housing and day centres reflect the changing patterns of treatment for mental ill-health. Effects of long-term institutionalisation, which may lead to deterioration in motivation and personal care, will be increasingly evident in the community as hospitals close and financial support for community care is not forthcoming.

12.2 Oral health and disease

With advances in treatment, particularly the development of medication that controls or reduces the effect of symptoms, there is evidence to suggest that individuals on long-term psychiatric medication are more at risk of oral disease.[6-9] Depending on the diagnosis, medication may often have to be taken for life.

A study comparing oral health in a matched sample of individuals, with and without chronic mental illness living in the community, confirms the risk factors.[10] The primary factor was considered to be the mental disorder, while associated factors were financial constraints, lifestyle and poor oral hygiene. The side-effect of psychotropic medication in reducing salivary secretions was an additional, important factor.

Dry mouth was a consistent feature of the group with mental illness. Dental caries of the smooth surfaces of teeth and root surfaces (mainly seen in the older population) was higher in the sample with mental illness than in the control group, possibly due to an increased consumption of carbonated drinks (*Colour Plates* **8, 9**) reported by the mentally ill. Periodontal disease was also more severe.

The side-effects of many of the major psychiatric drugs are highlighted in the literature; their oral side-effects are summarised in *Table 12.1*. Poor compliance has justified the use of sustained-release medication, which can be administered by tablet or injection at intervals of up to a month. While advances in psychiatric medication have had a significant impact on the treatment and prognosis of mental illness, the prescription of long-term medication without informing the individual of the range of possible side-effects has been raised and questioned by MIND.[11] There does not

Table 12.1 Oral and facial side-effects of antipsychotic medication.*

Drug	*Side-effects*
Antidepressants	
Tricyclic antidepressants	Dry mouth
	Involuntary facial movements
Monoamine oxidase inhibitors	Dry mouth
Hypnotics	
Promethazine hydrochloride	Dry mouth
Anxiolytics	
Chlormezanone	Dry mouth
Hydroxyzine hydrochloride	Dry mouth
Anti-psychotic drugs	
Phenothiazines	Involuntary facial movement
Butyrophenones	Dry mouth
	Involuntary facial movements
Anti-manic drugs	
Lithium	Dry mouth
Carbamazepine	Involuntary facial movements
Anti-parkinsonian drugs	Dry mouth

* Source: *British National Formulary*. September 1991, No. 22.

People Suffering from Mental Illness

appear to be any documented evidence to show that, if information is given, this also includes advice on the oral side-effects or the implications for oral health, and that appropriate counselling is given by health professionals.

The side-effects of major psychiatric drugs may be relatively unimportant to an individual compared to the potential for relief of psychiatric symptoms. However, the implications of oral side-effects in oral and dental disease need to be highlighted.

Attention to oral hygiene, prevention and diet is essential, together with regular dental attendance to advise, monitor and treat, if oral side-effects are to be minimised. This chapter will concentrate on the commoner psychiatric conditions and their potential for oral disease.

12.3 Barriers to oral health

Illness, whether physical or mental, leads to a deterioration in self-care. Important factors include a lack of motivation and a temporary or permanent loss of ability, knowledge and skill. Oral care may already have a low priority, and in certain phases of an individual's illness may have an even lower priority or be non-existent.

Traditional barriers to dental care which apply to the total population[12] will also apply to the non-homogeneous proportion who may be suffering from mental illness. Socio-economic factors, life-style, personality changes and psychological factors which affect 'normal function' may interfere with relationships. The individual's moods and behaviour or inability to function 'normally' may act as additional barriers to self-care and to seeking help and treatment, including dental treatment (*Table 12.2*).

Table 12.2 Behavioural factors in mental illness

Impaired ability to learn	Anxiety
Deterioration in personal care	Fear
Poor motivation	Delusions
Amnesia	Hallucinations
Disorientation	Paranoia
Mood changes	

12.4 Side-effects of medication

Most of the major drugs used to alleviate or control psychiatric symptoms have side-effects. The most commonly used medications are:

165

Holistic Oral Care

- Tranquillisers.
- Long-acting tranquillisers.
- Tricyclic antidepressants.
- Monoamine oxidase inhibitors (MAOIs).
- Lithium and its derivatives.
- Anti-parkinsonian drugs.

Side-effects may be physiological and produce other behavioural symptoms or mood changes. Those side-effects that may affect oral health are summarised in *Table 12.1*.

The most common oral side-effect of psychiatric medication is a dry mouth (xerostomia) caused by reduced salivary secretion. The implications of dry mouth as a factor in increasing the risks of dental caries, periodontal disease and oral infections were described in Chapter 2. Signs, symptoms, and the treatment of dry mouth are summarised in *Table 12.3*. Other side-effects which affect mood may influence oral care, and involuntary facial movements make dental treatment difficult for both patient and clinician.

Table 12.3 Dry mouth (xerostomia)

Signs and symptoms	*Management*
Dry mouth	Improve oral hygiene
Difficulty with speech	Chlorhexidine gel or mouthwash
swallowing	Avoid sugar-sweetened drinks
dentures	Frequent sips of iced water
Disturbed taste sensation	Suck chips of ice
Increased caries rate	Evian atomised spray
Increased periodontal disease	Saliva substitutes
Oral infections	Refer to doctor or dentist for advice
Salivary gland infections	Refer to doctor or dentist for advice

12.5 Neuroses

Neuroses are disorders of emotional or intellectual functioning which do not deprive the individual of contact with reality. These may be further classified as:

- Personality disorders.
- Anxiety and phobic states.
- Hysterical states.
- Obsessive–compulsive disorders.
- Grief and neurotic depression.

Personality disorders

There are no specific oral problems associated with personality disorders, although some behavioural characteristics may create barriers to seeking dental care. Sensitive and skilled handling by the dental team is necessary to establish a good relationship. Irregular dental attendance and frequent changes of dentist are the likely consequence of a poor relationship between patient and dental team. The oral side-effects of medication used to control behaviour must be considered in relation to oral health.

Anxiety and phobias

Anxiety states commonly occur in psychiatric disorders. Fear and anxiety, often amounting to panic, characterise this unwelcome state. Among the classic features of 'flight and fight', caused by the action of the sympathetic autonomic nervous system, are the common symptoms of increased anxiety, hypertension, alertness, loss of appetite and dry mouth.

Dentists are familiar with anxiety as a daily feature of dental practice. In many cases, this is a learnt response from parents and family or is due to previous unpleasant or traumatic dental experiences.[13-15] Fear of, and anxiety about, dentistry has a direct influence on the attendance patterns of these individuals, who mainly seek dental care for the relief of pain. Dental phobics are reported to suffer pain for an average of 17.3 days before attending a dental clinic as compared with non-phobics with an average of 3.0 days' delay in attendance.[15]

Non-attendance leads to lack of, or delayed, treatment. Without resorting to treatment under a general anaesthetic or intravenous sedation, completely pain-free treatment may be impossible, thus reinforcing and justifying the original fear. Tooth loss may be inevitable. The use of hostility by individuals to mask their fear in the dental situation creates a communication barrier between patient and clinician, which may further reinforce barriers.

Specific phobias which interfere with 'normal' daily living may also act as barriers to dental care. Needle phobics need support in obtaining appropriate treatment to enable them to overcome their problem. Increasingly, desensitisation, relaxation techniques and hypnosis are being used by the dental profession to help such patients.

People who suffer from agoraphobia and who are confined to their own home are isolated from information and services. There is clearly a need for local information on available domiciliary dental services to be made known to this group and their carers. This could be achieved by an out-reach approach to professional and voluntary agencies involved in identifying and supporting agoraphobics.

Hysterical neuroses

There are no demonstrable oral problems associated with hysterical states, although a number of physical complaints without a demonstrable organic cause have been reported.[16] These may affect the oral cavity and include:

Holistic Oral Care

- Pain.
- Anaesthesia.
- Delusional halitosis.
- Dysphagia.
- Cancerophobia.

It is important that oral complaints are investigated by referral for a dental opinion. This provides the opportunity to eliminate oral disease as a cause of the complaint and to provide reassurance where necessary.

Obsessional neuroses

These may rarely be centred on the mouth and may include compulsive toothbrushing, the excessive use of mouthwashes or obsession with the possibility of oral infection.[16] If there is an obsession with maintaining oral hygiene, rigorous oral care using incorrect or over-vigorous toothbrushing techniques may lead to enamel abrasion and recession of the gingival margins.

A high rate of psychiatric disorder (80%) has been reported in patients attending a specialist pain clinic.[17] In a study of self-reported halitosis subjects in Nigeria, all subjects with no previous history of drug abuse or psychiatric treatment were considered to be suffering from delusional halitosis.[18] Dental advice or treatment may be sought repeatedly as a means of reinforcing or confirming an obsession, and referral for psychiatric assessment may be initiated by the dentist.

Depressive neuroses

Reactive or neurotic depression, which is characterised by mental withdrawal and a lowered mood, may be an over-reaction to 'normal' loss as in grief, or as a response to physical illness or a major change in life circumstances. Neurotic depressive illness is reported to occur most often in young adults as a reaction to stress.[19]

General apathy, loss of appetite and sleep disturbances, together with periods of anxiety or agitation, may lead inevitably to a deterioration in self-care. Depression has also been associated with a number of orofacial complaints[20]:

- Atypical facial pain.
- Burning mouth.
- Sore tongue.
- Pain and dysfunction of the temporomandibular joint.
- Oral delusions.
- Dry mouth.
- Spots or lumps.
- Excessive salivary secretion.
- Disturbances of taste sensation.

Some of the above may be directly attributed to the side-effects of medication. The drugs most commonly used for the treatment of depression are the monoamine oxidase inhibitors and tricyclic antidepressants. Both produce a dry mouth, which is particularly notable in the tricyclics which have a strong anticholinergic effect. Dry mouth is reported to be less of a problem in the newer tricyclic drugs. In a study involving 47 patients with burning mouth syndrome, more than half were considered to have a psychological component to their complaint[21]. A dental opinion should be sought to eliminate oral disease and to establish a programme for oral health and prevention which minimises the effect of reduced salivary secretion.

Temporomandibular joint pain may be associated with compulsive or stress-related habits, such as clenching, chewing, or grinding (bruxism). Loss of the molar teeth is a common contributory factor in this condition, and the provision of dentures to replace missing teeth and restore the occlusion may produce relief. Soft splints or bite-guards which cover the teeth may also provide relief and prevent recurrent habits. Analgesics, muscle relaxants and mild anxiolytics may be prescribed for the relief of pain.

12.6 Psychoses

Psychoses are defined as illnesses where individuals, in the acute phase, are out of touch with reality. They are characterised by a profound and essential disturbance in the individual's appreciation of the nature of their environment and their response to it. They are classified into four major groups:

- Affective disorder: psychotic depression,
   mania.
- Organic cerebral disorders: delirium,
   epilepsy,
   dementia.
- Disorders of old age.
- Schizophrenia.

Psychotic depression
This is considered to be a pathological condition characterised by acute misery, malaise and despair which grossly exceed a 'normal' response to the precipitating loss or crisis.

In some cases, it occurs spontaneously and the individual has a distorted view of reality, with delusions and, in some cases, hallucinations. Involutional melancholia describes depressive illness in the age group 45 to 65; in women, this is accompanied by agitation and may be associated with the menopause.

Familial tendencies, stress, neurochemistry and the stressful effects of debilitating physical illness, particularly endocrine disorders, are considered to be aetiological factors. It occurs commonly as a secondary feature of other psychiatric conditions, such as schizophrenia, anxiety states and alcoholism. Cognitive theories view psychotic depression as a syndrome of aggression turned inwardly against the self.

Mood changes, generalised withdrawal, apathy and inertia, agitation, anxiety, fatigue and physiological disturbances in sleep, appetite and digestion have an inevitable effect on self-care. Oral care may have no importance in such a distressing and gloomy, even suicidal, state of mind. Treatment is with a combination of antidepressants and symptomatic drugs, together with supportive psychotherapy and electroconvulsive therapy. The major drugs used for the treatment of psychotic depression are:

- Tricyclic antidepressants.
- Tetracyclic antidepressants.
- Bicyclic antidepressants.
- Monoamine oxidase inhibitors (MAOIs).
- Combination drugs.

A dry mouth is a consistent side-effect of the cyclic antidepressants. Reduced salivary secretion is also a side-effect of the MAOIs and a potential side-effect of combination antidepressives which contain major tranquillisers. Major tranquillisers cause 'tardive dyskinesia', which describes distinctive involuntary and repetitive movements of the facial muscles. However, these are unlikely to occur with the small doses of major tranquillisers found in combination drugs.

Certain antipsychotic drugs which have antidepressant properties, such as flupenthixol, tryptophan and fluvoxamine, are reported to have fewer side-effects and are less likely to reduce salivary secretion.

Manic psychosis

Manic disorders are often referred to as bipolar disorders, as characteristic periods of extreme elation and irritability are frequently associated with depressive episodes. During the manic phase task-orientated attention is lacking, while during the depressive phase motivation and drive are absent. These disorders are reported to first occur in young adults, whereas in the elderly they may indicate organic disease or be secondary to the effect of drugs.

The prognosis for treatment of the manic phase has dramatically improved with the use of lithium, which is reported to occasionally cause a dry mouth. Antidepressive medication may be prescribed during the depressive phase. Interaction with antipsychotics, such as droperidol, may cause facial dyskinesias, which are distressing to the patient and pose management problems for dental treatment.

People Suffering from Mental Illness

Lithium may precipitate cardiac arrhythmias, which pose a risk for general anaesthesia; lithium treatment may therefore need to be discontinued a few days before a general anaesthetic is given. Preventive oral hygiene to avoid the need for a dental general anaesthetic is important.

Friedlander and Birch[22] carried out an interesting study in Los Angeles on the dental condition of patients with bipolar disorder on long-term lithium therapy. During the depressive phase, most subjects with natural teeth (85%) had severe gingivitis with extensive visible deposits of plaque and calculus. Total disregard for proper oral hygiene was noted. Three subjects reported a generalised stomatitis which occurred each time lithium therapy was recommenced.

Dry mouth was reported in 78% of subjects, with a few reporting a burning sensation in the lips and tongue, difficulty with speech, and changes in taste sensation. The subjects' response to dry mouth (xerostomia) was mostly an increased consumption of 'candy' and drinks with a high sugar content to relieve thirst – behaviour which predisposes to dental caries.

During the manic phase of the illness, a dry mouth was not a problem but subjects reported that it had been a problem during depressive phases. The sample in the manic phase was too small to draw conclusive comparisons. However, the authors concluded that the dental condition in the subjects studied appeared to be a function of their emotional state and its influence both on salivary flow and poor oral hygiene. In those individuals who increased their intake of cariogenic food and drink, the potential for oral and dental disease was greater.

Further research is needed to identify the relevant importance of attention, motivation and drive in the manic and depressive phases, changes in salivary flow during the depressive phase, and the oral side-effects of medication. Dietary counselling and advice on improving oral hygiene should be a priority, as well as advice on management of a dry mouth and the use of saliva substitutes. Changes in life-style may be more difficult to achieve but regular dental attendance should be encouraged in people with manic depression.

Organic cerebral disorders
Organic brain disease may underlie physical symptoms of delirium, epilepsy and dementia.

Delirium
Personal care is likely to be poor in delirium, which is characterised by a clouding of consciousness, recent memory failure, and a failure of attention, concentration and judgement. Thus the individual will be highly dependent on others for personal and oral care. Disturbed behaviour may be controlled with chlorpromazine, haloperidol or thioridazine, all of which reduce salivary secretions.

Dementia

Dementia is defined as 'organic loss of intellectual functioning' and is the result of deterioration in previously normal brain function. It is global in that it affects all faculties in a previously alert individual, and is generally considered to be irreversible. Onset occurs primarily in later life and is relatively uncommon below the age of 60. Approximately 5% of the population over 65 and 20% aged 80 years and over are estimated to suffer from dementia. About half suffer from Alzheimer's disease, 15% from cerebrovascular dementia, 20% from both, and approximately 15% from other mainly degenerative conditions. Aetiological factors are given in *Table 12.4*.

Table 12.4 Aetiological factors in dementia.

Type of dementia	Aetiology
Primary degenerative brain disease	Alzheimer's disease Pick's disease Huntington's chorea Creutzfeldt–Jakob syndrome
Cerebrovascular disease	Atherosclerotic (multi-infarct) dementia
Dementia secondary to other conditions	Brain injury Anoxic brain damage Infection Poisoning Metabolic and endocrine disorders Neoplasms Hydrocephalus Epilepsy

Alzheimer's disease, also called senile and presenile dementia, is the commonest type of dementia. Necrotic areas of the cerebral cortex were first described by Alzheimer in 1906. The identification of biochemical brain changes, in particular a decrease in the levels of acetylcholine transferase, have prompted research into new drug treatments.

The first sign is often an exaggerated loss of memory for recent events, which progresses with confusion, loss of language function and memory failure to dementia. Behavioural problems and severe dementia develop in the later stages. The course of the disease is variable and may be aggravated by isolation, sensory deprivation, physical illness, the side-effects of medication, and by family pressures and tensions.

Genetic factors are increasingly recognised as playing a role in Alzheimer's disease, although other factors are involved. Specific genetic defects have been identified on chromosome 21 (the abnormal chromosome in Down's syndrome), which is involved in the formation of excessive amounts of a protein found in the brains of Alzheimer's subjects. In the rare familial form of the disease, autosomal-dominant inheritance has been identified. Studies which link Alzheimer's disease with aluminium have provided a new avenue for research.

There is no treatment which significantly reverses or slows down the progress of the disease, although there have been some encouraging results using drugs which act by increasing levels of acetylcholine in the brain. Drugs currently in use are physostigmine, THA and HP029. Acetyl-L-carnitine has also been tried with some success. Drugs that facilitate the elimination of aluminium from the body are under trial in Canada and are showing some promising results. In new drug trials, oral side-effects should be noted.

Both Pick's disease and Creutzfeldt–Jakob syndrome are rare forms of degenerative brain disease. Pick's disease mainly affects the frontal and parietal lobes. Creutzfeldt–Jakob syndrome is caused by a virus and is characterised by progressive dementia and sometimes muscle wasting, tremor, athetosis and spastic dysarthria.

Huntington's chorea is well-known as a hereditary disease which appears mainly in middle age. It is characterised by involuntary movements and dementia. The involuntary movements and an inability to co-operate affect oral care and treatment. Some antiparkinsonian drugs which reduce salivary secretions may be prescribed to control involuntary movements.

Atherosclerotic dementia
In this condition, multiple small haemorrhages and infarcts caused by atherosclerosis of the cranial arteries result in localised areas of brain damage. Depression, mood swings and a tendency to weep are more typical of this type of dementia. Antidepressants used to control the depressive aspects of this condition may reduce salivary flow.

Other forms of dementia
The main causes are described earlier in this section. The underlying cause of dementia, the effects of mental decline, medication and deteriorating personal care on the individual's oral health must be considered. Other causes include human immune deficiency virus (HIV) infection, which is an increasing cause of dementia affecting younger people. The oral aspects of HIV and acquired immunodeficiency syndrome (AIDS) are discussed in detail in Chapter 14. It is important that carers are made aware of the predominant oral infections which occur and the techniques for managing oral care in a sensible, safe and practical way.

Deep ulcers affecting the skin and oral tissues, which may progress to destroy the underlying bone, are a feature of neurosyphilis. The most significant oral symptom in neurosyphilis is leukoplakia (*Colour Plate 27*), a condition characterised by thick white patches which occur particularly on the surface of the tongue. These lesions have a high potential for malignant change. Syphilitic cardiovascular disease may affect the management of dental treatment.

Holistic Oral Care

Oral problems in dementia

Memory loss, confusion and an impaired ability to perform perceptuo-motor skills lead to neglect and deterioration in personal care. Oral health will be affected, and personal and oral care will be the responsibility of a carer in most cases. A study of older people living in the community and suffering from the early stages of dementia demonstrated poor levels of oral and denture hygiene[23]; 92% had no natural teeth as compared with 87% of the control group. Dentures worn by the mentally ill were significantly older than those in the control group and 76% of the mentally ill had not visited the dentist in the previous six years as compared with 58% of the control group. These findings should be viewed in relation to the oral status and dental attendance patterns of older people, many of whom are themselves carers (Chapter 4).

The provision of counselling on oral care to carers and dental attendance is necessary in the early stages of the disease to prevent oral pathology and to provide treatment while the individual is still able to communicate and co-operate. The individual's ability to adjust to new dentures decreases with their ability to co-operate. The effects of anticonvulsant therapy for the treatment of epilepsy may also need to be considered. The risk of oral disease is increased by the use of anticholinergic drugs to treat depression, involuntary movements and other medical conditions, as such drugs will reduce salivary flow.

The burden of responsibility and care for the elderly mentally ill rests mainly with the family as approximately 80% live in their own or in a close relative's home.[24] Family carers are most often wives or daughters who suffer considerable personal and emotional hardship, coping with a relative whose condition is inevitably going to deteriorate, and in many cases with little or no support from statutory services.

In a postal survey of carers identified through the Alzheimer's Disease Society[25], 96% felt that dental care was important; 53% cared for a dependent who had natural teeth and, of these, 51% reported dental problems in the previous year. Oral problems were reported in 39% of Alzheimer sufferers who had no natural teeth. The inability to ascertain whether an Alzheimer's patient is in pain was reported as very distressing to one carer. Comments on the dental profession's lack of awareness of the problems of dementia suggest the need for greater interdisciplinary training and co-operation.

Approximately half the carers felt that dental care was best provided in a dental surgery, although comments were made about 'disorientation' and 'waiting times'. Domiciliary dental care was less popular except for older dependants with no teeth. This may have been due to the carers' lack of knowledge about portable dental equipment which can be set up in the home. The importance of familiar surroundings in reducing disorientation may make domiciliary dental care more popular with carers if they were better informed about the type of dental care which can be provided at home.

Health professionals have an important role in counselling and informing carers of risks to oral health, providing preventive advice and facilitating contact with a suitable and sympathetic source of dental care.

Schizophrenia

Historically, schizophrenia was thought to be an expression of 'split personality', epitomising the concept of 'madness' – a view which is still upheld and sensationalised by ignorance and misuse of the term. Originally called 'dementia praecox', schizophrenia is now accepted as the term for a group of severe emotional disorders, which are characterised by a progressive disintegration of the individual's personality and a psychological detachment from the real world. Symptoms include misinterpretation and retreat from reality, delusions, hallucinations, indifference, inappropriate moods, withdrawn and sometimes bizarre, or regressive, behaviour.[26] The accuracy of schizophrenia as a diagnostic psychiatric label has been challenged by Laing and Esterson[27], who analysed a number of diagnosed cases in relation to family and social influences.

The significance of inherited aspects is now accepted, while neurochemical or metabolic abnormalities, social adjustment, unresolved interpersonal psychological conflicts and faulty child/parent relationships are all factors now considered to be relevant and significant.[28] With such a wide and culturally defined concept of 'schizophrenia and schizophrenic-type illness', as well as variations in survey methodology, it is not surprising that there are variable demographic prevalence rates.[29] Nevertheless, it is reported to affect approximately 1% of the world population with national variations due to different diagnostic criteria. A wider concept of the schizophrenic personality is estimated to occur in some 3% of the population, characterised by social and personal withdrawal, sometimes with eccentricity, shyness and reticence, hypersensitivity and suspicious tendencies.

The onset of schizophrenia is usually in early adulthood and generally appears about 10 years earlier in males than in females. Differences occur in the acute and chronic phases of schizophrenia. In the acute phase, symptoms may include hallucinations, delusions and thought disorder, and in the chronic phase, flattening of emotion, social withdrawal and reduced verbal communication. No two cases are identical and the reader is advised to consult other sources for a greater understanding of this complex and disabling illness.

There are no specific oral or dental problems related to schizophrenia. However, oral delusions such as teeth being 'bugged' or fitted with 'transmitters' have been encountered by the authors in some psychiatric in-patients. In one case, six anterior crowns were very neatly removed by a patient using a pair of electrical pliers; it was difficult to convince the patient that the temporary crowns fitted as a replacement had not been tampered with. Drugs which control hallucinations, reduce severe thought disorders and delusions and have a calming effect, have dramatically changed the outcome for sufferers. Behaviour becomes less antisocial, thus facilitating the individual's integration into society. A significant feature of schizophrenia is that the individual may have little insight into their illness and therefore compliance in taking regular antipsychotic medication may be poor.

Medication is usually taken for life with long-acting depot preparations given orally or by injection helping to overcome non-compliance. The drugs most commonly used in the treatment of schizophrenia are phenothiazines and butyrophenones. The tranquillising effect of these drugs is of secondary importance to their effect in controlling delusional symptoms. Many side-effects are reported, including dry mouth and tardive dyskinesia (involuntary facial and bodily movements). The latter may be irreversible. Parkinsonian side-effects include:

- Mask-like facial appearance due to stiff and weak muscles.
- Hand tremor.
- Pill-rolling movement of the fingers.
- Restlessness.
- Forward-leaning and shuffling gait.

Side-effects vary depending on the dose, duration, the particular drug used, and individual susceptibility. Haloperidol is reported to have less effect on salivary secretions; however, the other side-effects described above are more common.

Management of dental treatment may be more difficult in the acute phase and if tardive dyskinesia or parkinsonian features are present. While the management of schizophrenic symptoms must be the priority, every effort should be made to encourage good oral care and dietary control of sugars to reduce the oral health risks of a dry mouth.

Psychosis in older people

Almost all psychiatric disorders increase with age and reach a peak in old age. Some disorders represent the chronic state of earlier diagnosed disease. The most characteristic are:

- Delusional states.
- Depression.
- Dementia of organic origin.
- Paraphrenia (schizophrenia of late onset).
- Neurotic symptoms.
- Personality deterioration.

The causes have largely been covered in earlier sections of this chapter. Severe depressive reactions may occur as a consequence of ageing and loss – such as bereavement, loneliness, progressive disability and an impoverishment in the quality of life – to name but a few. Loss of memory, sensory impairment, a lack of social contact and social isolation contribute

People Suffering from Mental Illness

to paranoid states. Physical illness may be associated with delusions. A diagnosis of paranoid schizophrenia is only made when there is evidence of personality deterioration.

Treatment with medication has variable results, partly due to memory loss and non-compliance. Doses are generally lower, but drug interactions must be considered and side-effects may be more pronounced. Dry mouth may be potentiated by multiple prescribing with antipsychotic medication, antihypertensives, antiemetics, decongestants and bronchodilators, to name just a few of the drugs which reduce salivary secretions. The effect of dryness on the thin atrophic soft tissues of the older person's mouth can be severely distressing. Good oral hygiene and saliva substitutes can provide some relief. Dental management is affected by behavioural aspects and multiple medication.

12.7 Psychosomatic disorders

In viewing health and illness holistically, it is evident that some illnesses will originate in the individual's 'mind'. The complex interaction of the various anatomical, physiological and biochemical systems is still poorly understood. Emotional responses, which are a combination of complex biophysiological changes and external experience, can lead an individual to believe that they are suffering from an imaginary illness, or pain which is subjectively real.

It is beyond the scope of this guide to explore this interesting topic in depth, but if an oral complaint is expressed then a dental opinion may be needed to eliminate oral pathology. Burning mouth, dry mouth, halitosis, disturbed taste sensations and oral or facial pain are the commonest complaints. Interdisciplinary assessment may be necessary to reach a diagnosis.

12.8 Anorexia nervosa and bulimia

These are eating disorders which are reported to affect mainly young females who have an obsession or phobia with weight gain and body image. However, these conditions are reported to be increasing in young males in Western society. The incidence increased fourfold from the mid-sixties to the late seventies and early eighties[30] in a climate of heightened cultural and social pressure to be slim.

In anorexia, the individual has a profound aversion to food which in extreme cases leads to starvation. Bulimia is characterised by over-eating, sometimes accompanied by self-induced or spontaneous vomiting. Bulimia is thought to be stress-related and bingeing often includes a high proportion of cariogenic food. Laxatives are sometimes taken to induce weight loss. Both conditions can co-exist or alternate in the same individual and may be regarded as hysterical conditions.

Holistic Oral Care

The objectives of treatment are to establish rapport, followed by nursing, dietary and supportive regimes to restore body weight, with therapy to deal with the underlying psychopathological disorders. There are no specific oral problems associated with eating disorders.

However, malnutrition, dehydration, symptomatic behaviour and drugs used in the treatment of anxiety or vomiting affect the mouth (*Table 12.5*). Anaemia may occur as a result of acute malnutrition and poses a risk for general anaesthesia and an increased susceptibility to infection. The parotid salivary glands may be enlarged and angular cheilitis, soreness and inflammation at the angle of the mouth caused by candidal infection may occur.

Table 12.5 Oral symptoms in eating disorders.

Enlargement of the parotid salivary glands
Erosion of the teeth due to persistent vomiting
Angular cheilitis
Sore throat due to vomiting
Anaemia
Ulcers due to accidental trauma to induce vomiting

Tooth erosion (Chapter 2) due to acid regurgitation affecting the palatal, lingual and occlusal surfaces of the teeth is a commonly reported dental disorder (*Colour Plate* **13**).[31] Immediate or excessive toothbrushing after vomiting may account for excessive wear of tooth surfaces. Ulcers in the area of the pharynx due to accidental trauma to induce vomiting are also reported. Some antiemetics prescribed to control vomiting reduce salivary secretion.

With regular dental attendance, a dentist may be the first to make a provisional diagnosis of an eating disorder, particularly when a thin young female presents with erosion of the palatal and lingual surfaces of the teeth. Preventive advice and treatment for the oral effects include:

- Fluoride toothpaste.
- Fluoride mouthwash.
- Topical fluoride professionally applied.
- Splints to protect teeth during vomiting.

Professional treatment may also be required for angular cheilitis or oral trauma.

12.9 Alcohol and substance abuse

Substance use, abuse and dependence is increasing. The high incidence of HIV infection amongst intravenous drug users has raised the profile of substance abuse in health-promotion targeting. Psychiatric illness is reported in both alcoholism and in the use of illicit drugs. Personal neglect may also be a feature.

Blackouts, hallucinations, delirium tremens following withdrawal, Korsakoff's syndrome and alcoholic dementia summarise the psychiatric problems associated with alcoholism. Oral problems encountered in alcoholism are usually due to personal neglect and poor oral hygiene and include:

- Advanced dental caries.
- Periodontal disease.
- Angular cheilitis.
- Oral signs of anaemia.

Other problems arise due to accidental maxillofacial injury and trauma. Medical conditions associated with alcohol abuse may affect general health and seriously affect the individual's suitability for a general anaesthetic. The incidence of oral cancer in alcohol and tobacco users is discussed in Chapters 1 and 2.

Addiction to narcotics and other substances is a complex subject. Psychiatric disorders may be a result of addiction or withdrawal, or of the use of hallucinogenic drugs. Solvent abuse, which mainly occurs in the early teens, may lead to paranoid or aggressive outbursts.

There are few specific oral problems associated with these groups other than those which are due to personal oral neglect. Dental caries and periodontal disease are increased in cocaine addiction, while lesions around the mouth have been noted in solvent abuse. Dental treatment may be more difficult to provide due to withdrawal, and to behavioural changes, and may be affected by compromised general health.

There is an increased risk of HIV infection and hepatitis B carrier status in intravenous drug users (Chapter 14). Gloves should be worn by anyone carrying out oral hygiene on known carriers and people who fall into high-risk categories for carrier status.

12.10 People with learning disabilities

Psychiatric and behavioural disorders affect this group as they do the general population. The rate of psychiatric disorder is higher in a few syndromes which occur amongst the most profoundly handicapped. Oral and dental aspects are covered in depth in Chapter 11.

12.11 Children and adolescents

The aetiology of psychiatric disease in children and adolescents is complex and multi-factorial. Children may suffer from the effects of mental illness by default if a parent suffers from mental illness. Behavioural problems and stress-related psychiatric disorders do not of themselves produce any oral problems. Chronic or life-threatening illness may have an oral component, while behavioural problems may interfere with dental care. Behaviour which maintains oral health is most effective when established at an early age. The reader should refer to Chapter 3 for the principles of oral care and preventive advice for children.

12.12 Summary

The object of this chapter has been to highlight the oral and dental problems which are associated with the different categories of mental illness. It is clear that life-style, poor motivation, impaired mental function and disturbed or psychotic behaviour have an impact on oral health. The situation is complicated by the oral side-effects of antipsychotic medication, in particular the many drugs which reduce salivary secretion.

As the search continues for drugs with fewer side-effects, hopefully it will be possible to eliminate those of an anticholinergic nature that produce a reduction in saliva. With greater understanding of mental illness and an increased trend towards talking therapies, the prescription of medication may decrease. The role of health care professionals is paramount in ensuring that oral and dental problems are identified, and that appropriate advice and oral care are provided and support is given to make appropriate contact with dental services.

12.13 References

1. Thompson, D. and Pudney, M. (1990). *Mental Illness: The Fundamental Facts*. London, Mental Health Foundation.
2. Myers, J.K., Weissman, M.M. and Tischler, G.L. *et al.* (1984). Six-month prevalence of psychiatric disorders in three communities. *Archives of General Psychiatry*, **41**, 959–967.
3. Robins, L.N. *et al.* (1984). Lifetime prevalence of specific psychiatric disorders in three sites. *Archives of General Psychiatry*, **41**, 949–958.
4. Miniszek, N.A. (1983). Development of Alzheimer's disease in Down's syndrome individuals. *American Journal of Mental Deficiency*, **87**(4), 377–385.
5. Stafford-Clark, D., Bridges, P. and Black, D. (1990). *Psychiatry for Students*. 7th ed. London, Unwin Hyman, pp. 141–142.
6. Rundegren, J. *et al.* (1985). Oral conditions in patients receiving long-term treatment with cyclic antidepressants. *Swed. Dent. J.*, **9**, 55–64.
7. Slome, B.A. (1984). Rampant caries: a side-effect of tricyclic antidepressant therapy. *Gen. Dent.*, **32**, 494–495.
8. Bassuk, E., and Schoonover, S. (1978). Rampant dental caries in the treatment of depression. *J. Clin. Psychiatry*, **39**, 163–165.

9. Winer, J.A. and Bahn, S. (1967). Loss of teeth with antidepressant therapy. *Arch. Gen. Psychiatry*, **16**, 239–240.
10. Stiefel, D.J. *et al*. (1990). A comparison of the oral health of persons with and without chronic mental illness in community settings. *Spec. Care in Dent.*, Jan–Feb, 6–12.
11. MIND. (1990). *People First. Special Report*. MIND/Roehampton People First Survey. London, MIND.
12. Finch, H., Keegan, J., Ward, K. and Sen, B.S. (1988). *Barriers to the receipt of dental care – a qualitative study*. London: Social and Community Planning Research.
13. Shaw, O. (1975). Dental anxiety in children. *Br. Dent. J.*, **139**, 134–139.
14. Fogione, A.L. and Clarke, R.E. (1974). Comments on an empirical study of the causes of dental fears. *J. Dent. Res.*, **53**, 496.
15. Lautch, H.A. (1971). Dental phobia. *Br. J. Psychiatry*, **119**, 151–158.
16. Scully, C. and Cawson, A. (1987). *Medical Problems in Dentistry*. 2nd ed. Bristol, Wright, pp. 393.
17. Hughes, A.M. *et al*. (1989). Psychiatric disorders in a dental clinic. *Br. Dent. J.*, **166**, 16–19.
18. Iwu, C.O. and Akpata, O. (1989). Delusional halitosis. Review of the literature and analysis of 32 cases. *Br. Dent. J.*, **167**, 294–296.
19. Stafford-Clark, D., Bridges, P. and Black, D. (1990). *Psychiatry for Students*. 7th ed. London, Unwin Hyman, pp. 89–90.
20. Scully, C. and Cawson, A. (1987). *Medical Problems in Dentistry*. 2nd ed. Bristol, Wright, pp. 385–386.
21. Lamb, A.B., Lamey, P.J. and Reeve, P.E. (1988). Burning mouth syndrome: psychological aspects. *Br. Dent. J.*, **165**, 256–260.
22. Friedlander, A.H. and Birch, N.J. (1990). Dental conditions in patients with bipolar disorder on long-term lithium. *Spec. Care in Dent.*, Sept–Oct, pp. 148–149.
23. Whittle, J.G., Grant, A.A. and Worthington, H.V. (1987). The dental health of the elderly mentally ill: a preliminary report. *Br. Dent. J.*, **162**, 381–383.
24. O'Donovan, S. (1991). The support needs of those caring for elderly mentally infirm relatives. (Editorial.) *Signpost*. Cardiff, South Glamorgan Service Development Team (EMI), **18**(8), 1–2.
25. Whittle, J.G., Grant, A.A. and Worthington, H.V. (1988). The dental health of the elderly mentally ill: the carers' perspective. *Br. Dent. J.*, **164**, 144–147.
26. *Dorland's Illustrated Medical Dictionary*. 26th ed. Philadelphia, W.B. Saunders.
27. Laing, R.D. and Esterson, A. (1964). *Sanity, Madness and the Family*. Middlesex, Penguin Books.
28. Stafford-Clark, D., Bridges, P. and Black, D. (1990). *Psychiatry for Students*. 7th ed. London, Unwin Hyman, p. 138.
29. Shur, E. (1988). The epidemiology of schizophrenia. *Br. J. Hosp. Med.*, **40**, 38–45.
30. Szumkler, G.I. (1985). The incidence of anorexia nervosa and bulimia. *J. Psychiatr. Res.*, **19**, 143–154.
31. Milosevic, A. and Slade, P.D. (1989). The orodental status of anorexics and bulimics. *Br. Dent. J.*, **167**, 66–70.

13 Medically Compromised Patients

13. 1 Introduction
13. 2 Cardiovascular disease
13. 3 Blood disorders (dyscrasias)
13. 4 Bleeding disorders
13. 5 Respiratory disorders
13. 6 Gastrointestinal disease
13. 7 Liver disease
13. 8 Kidney disease
13. 9 Diabetes
13.10 Summary
13.11 References

13.1 Introduction

Whereas earlier chapters in Section 3 have covered oral health in three disability areas, both this and the next two chapters concentrate on medical conditions which may affect oral health. They are therefore slightly more technical than earlier chapters. Oral disease and discomfort may be the direct result of illness or secondary to its treatment. Conditions where general health is compromised by poor oral health are included. Furthermore, dental management may be complicated and pose a potential risk to health; dental treatment under general anaesthesia may pose a serious health risk. Preventive oral care, good oral hygiene and regular dental attendance to avoid crisis management are therefore a priority.

13.2 Cardiovascular diseases

Cardiovascular diseases are the commonest cause of death in industrialised society. They are also the commonest group of conditions which directly affect the provision of dental treatment. General anaesthesia for dental treatment in many cardiac conditions is best avoided and when necessary, managed in a hospital setting; it is perhaps one of the most important reasons for preventive oral hygiene and dental care. Anti-coagulant therapy clearly poses a risk of haemorrhage following dental extractions; dental

Medically Compromised Patients

treatment is therefore elective and carried out in consultation with the cardiologist and haematologist. The effect of anti-coagulant therapy on pro-thrombin times (INR) may need to be monitored and anticoagulant therapy adjusted prior to dental treatment. A number of cardiac conditions put the individual at risk of infective endocarditis.

Although there are few primary oral features, the side-effects of medication are an important consideration and the reader is advised to consult the latest *British National Formulary* or equivalent to identify possible oral side-effects related to specific drugs. Medication may affect dental management, particularly for dental treatment under general anaesthesia.

Historically, dental disease was thought to be the cause of certain cardiac conditions and extraction of the complete dentition was carried out to prevent cardiac infection from dental sepsis. Fortunately, this is no longer the case; however, the elimination of oral and dental infection as a potential cause of infective endocarditis remains a priority.

For the dental profession, a history of cardiac disease requires careful dental treatment planning. A detailed history which takes account of cardiac diagnosis and medication is paramount. If cognitive problems affect the accuracy of the medical history, then a medical examination and opinion will be requested to eliminate heart murmurs and other cardiac pathology. Dental treatment is planned to minimise stress and anxiety, under antibiotic cover if required, and with the avoidance of general anaesthesia if at all possible. Preventive oral care contributes to general health by reducing the need for, and the potential risks of, dental treatment. A team approach is essential.

Hypertension

There are no oral features associated with hypertension, although the avoidance of stress requires careful dental management. Some anti-hypertensives have a number of potential oral side-effects which are summarised in *Table 13.1*.

Table 13.1 Possible oral side-effects of anti-hypertensives.

Drug	Oral side-effects
Potassium-sparing diuretics	Dry mouth
Nifedipine (vasodilator)	Gingival hyperplasia
Beta blockers	White patches (lichenoid) Paraesthesia
Angiotensin inhibitors	Sore mouth or ulceration
Alpha blockers	White patches (lichenoid) or ulcers Dry mouth
Adrenergic neurone blockers	Dry mouth Pain in parotid salivary glands

Ischaemic heart disease
No specific oral features occur in ischaemic heart disease. However, dental management needs to be handled with care and treatment may have to be deferred until the patient's condition is stabilised. Pain in the jaw or oral tissues is a rare symptom of angina.

Anti-coagulants are frequently prescribed following by-pass surgery. Oral side-effects of drugs, particularly anti-hypertensives, must be considered (*Table 13.1*).

Cardiomyopathies
Diseases which affect the myocardium (muscles of the heart) are relatively uncommon apart from alcoholic heart muscle disease. Patients suffering from idiopathic cardiomyopathies are more at risk of infective endocarditis and at greater risk from general anaesthesia.

Cardiac arrhythmias
Patients suffering from cardiac arrythmias are a poor general anaesthetic risk. The effect of anti-coagulants and other cardiac medication must be considered. Patients with pacemakers should advise their dental practitioner so that contact with ultrasonic equipment which might affect the pacemaker's function can be avoided.

Rheumatic heart disease
Acute rheumatic fever (also called Sydenham's chorea and St. Vitus Dance when the illness is characterised by involuntary movements) poses a serious risk of subsequent chronic rheumatic heart disease. The prevalence of rheumatic heart disease has declined in industrialised society but remains a major health problem in developing countries.

Inflammation of cardiac tissues and in particular lasting damage to heart valves leads to chronic rheumatic heart disease which may be characterised by a heart murmur. This increases the risk of subsequent attacks of infective (bacterial) endocarditis caused by bacteria entering the blood stream. Dental treatment such as extractions and scaling is carried out under appropriate antibiotic cover for patients with a history of rheumatic heart disease.

Congenital heart disease
Cardiac defects caused by developmental abnormalities can be severely disabling, though the survival rate has improved with advances in cardiac surgery and antibiotics. Congenital heart disease is genetically determined in Down's syndrome (Chapter 11) and acquired in cases of rubella and cytomegaloviral infection. Other causes are not identified.

Oral features include delayed eruption of both primary and secondary teeth; this increases the possibility of malaligned teeth. Teeth may have a bluish tint, while caries and periodontal disease are reported to be more extensive, possibly due to poor oral hygiene and neglect.[1] Frequent prescription of sugar-based medicines in childhood may be a contributory factor. Higher levels of dental disease were demonstrated in a study of children with congenital heart disease, the majority of disease being found in children from poorer areas, and as a result a dental health education programme was developed for patients and their families attending cardiac outpatient clinics.[2]

Whatever the extent of cardiac damage, there is a risk of infective endocarditis following certain types of dental treatment. Bleeding tendencies and the risks of general anaesthesia are important factors in dental management. Dental care is managed in consultation with the cardiologist and provided under appropriate antibiotic cover.

Cardiac surgery and transplants

Advances in cardiac surgery for the repair and replacement of defective valves have improved life expectancy for many cardiac patients. Since dental sepsis was considered to be the major cause of infective endocarditis, pre-operative extractions of all teeth were carried out routinely. Fortunately, this is no longer considered to be necessary; close co-operation between cardiologist and the dental profession to ensure appropriate dental treatment, reducing the potential for oral infection before elective cardiac surgery, is becoming the norm. Antiseptic mouthwash, spray or gel may be prescribed to reduce levels of oral bacteria.

Post-operative anti-coagulant therapy affects dental management. Dental treatment for extraction and scaling is routinely carried out under antibiotic cover to protect against infective endocarditis.

Oral assessment and treatment with the prime objective of reducing the potential for oral infection is even more important prior to transplant surgery. Post-operative immunosuppression with drugs such as azothiaprine, cyclosporin, corticosteroids and antithymocyte globulin leads to a range of oral problems and increases the potential for opportunistic infections such as candidiasis (*Table 13.2*). Anticoagulant therapy is routine; aspirin and dipyridamole prolong the bleeding time.

Table 13.2 Oral side-effects of immunosuppression

Drug	*Oral side-effects*
Azothiaprine	Candidiasis
Antithymocyte globulin	Candidiasis
Corticosteroids	Candidiasis
Cyclosporin	Candidiasis
	Gingival hyperplasia

Infective (bacterial) endocarditis

There is a serious risk of infective endocarditis with a history of any type of heart lesion, and in particular defective or replacement heart valves.

Although extractions and scaling are considered to be a major risk, surveys have demonstrated that dental treatment precedes infection in approximately 10% of cases.[3] Host susceptibility, age, prosthetic heart valves, the level of oral infection and immunosupressive treatment are considered to be important predisposing factors.[4]

Bacteria may enter the blood stream from other procedures; arteriovenous shunts in renal disease and the release of intracranial pressure, intravenous medication and drug abuse, and cardiac catheterisation or cardiac surgery are cited.[4] However, antibiotic cover for dental treatment is used routinely as prophylaxis against infective endocarditis when the patient presents with a history of congenital or acquired valvular heart disease (*Table 13.3*).[5] Maintenance of oral health and regular dental attendance are recommended for those who are susceptible to infective endocarditis.

Table 13.3 Cardiac conditions at risk of infective endocarditis.

History of rheumatic fever	Coarctation of the aorta
Sydenham's chorea	Prosthetic heart valve
St. Vitus Dance	Degenerative valve disease
Ventricular septal defect	History of infective endocarditis
Patent ductus arteriosus	Repaired atrial septal defect
Persistent heart murmur	

Summary of risks

A summary of the risks associated with cardiovascular disease clearly demonstrates the importance of providing a full medical history prior to dental treatment. Professional collaboration is essential. Dental treatment may exacerbate anxiety and pain in cardiac conditions, general anaesthesia should be avoided or carried out under hospital conditions if necessary. Infective endocarditis is a serious dental management risk and the oral side-effects of medication may affect oral health and dental management. Preventive dental care reduces health risks and the need for dental intervention, thus maintaining oral health and comfort.

13.3 Blood disorders (dyscrasias)

Abnormalities in the number and type of red and white cells and platelets, and in the mechanisms for controlling bleeding, lead to a range of disorders. Anaemia due to a reduction in the amount of available haemoglobin in red cells is a symptom of underlying disease or blood loss. Bleeding disorders may be due to low platelet counts, prothrombin deficiency, deficiencies in clotting factors as in haemophilia, or secondary to anticoagulant therapy or drugs which depress bone marrow. Disorders of white cells whose primary role is bodily defence against infection lead to serious illness. Malignant blood disorders are described in Chapter 15.

Anaemia

Anaemia may be caused by one of a number of factors:

- Excessive haemorrhage.
- Abnormalities in red cell formation.
- Increased red cell destruction.

Underlying causes of anaemia are summarised in *Table 13.4*, and general oral features in *Table 13.5*.

Table 13.4 Causes of anaemia.

Excessive haemorrhage: menorrhagia
 gastro-intestinal ulcer/carcinoma
 trauma
Malabsorption syndromes
Pregnancy
Nutritional deficiencies
Drug induced anaemia
Leukaemia
Haemolytic anaemias
Secondary to drugs and chronic disease

Table 13.5 Oral signs and symptoms of anaemias.

Generalised soreness of soft tissues
Persistent ulceration
Red, smooth sore tongue (glossitis)
Candidal infection and angular cheilitis
Abnormalities in taste sensation

Oral symptoms are more common in anaemia due to iron, vitamin B_{12} or folic acid deficiency, whether caused by dietary deficiency or malabsorption. The tongue is particularly affected; oral candidal infection and angular cheilitis are common. Delayed healing affects dental management and reduced oxygen-carrying capacity of the blood poses a risk for general anaesthesia. Oral symptoms of underlying systemic disease must be considered.

Aplastic anaemia

Damage to bone marrow affects the number and quality of red cells. As well as the general symptoms of anaemia, additional factors which affect dental management include increased susceptibility to infection, bleeding tendencies, and the oral side-effects of corticosteroids. In Fanconi's anaemia, a rare genetic cause of aplastic anaemia, there may be a predisposition to oral carcinoma.[6]

Both aplastic anaemia and leukaemias may be treated by bone marrow transplantion, which leads to a range of distressing oral complaints. These are covered in greater depth in Chapter 15, on malignant disease.

Haemolytic anaemias

Causes of haemolytic anaemias include severe infection, septicaemia, drugs and chemicals, as well as hereditary factors. Malaria is the commonest global cause of the condition but is rare in the UK. General anaesthesia poses a major risk for dental management.

Congenital forms mainly affect certain racial groups. Sickle-cell disease occurs more frequently in subjects of African origin, but also in Asians and some Mediterranean groups.[7] Thalassaemias predominate in subjects of Middle Eastern, Asian or Mediterranean origin.[8]

Chronic susceptibility to infection affects oral health. Abnormalities affecting bone and teeth pose problems for dental management. Swollen parotid salivary glands and burning tongue are sometimes reported in the thalassaemias. However, the most important risk factor is in general anaesthesia. Preventive oral care, avoiding the need for dental intervention, is essential. Dental care when necessary is provided in consultation with the haematologist.

Leukaemias

These are covered in Chapter 15 on malignant disease. Acute oral infections and anaemia occur due to both the illness and its treatment.

13.4. Bleeding disorders

Bleeding disorders are caused by platelet or vascular disorders, anti-coagulant therapy or coagulation defects such as in haemophilia. In platelet disorders bleeding may be controlled by cortico-steroids, and in thrombocytopaenia, cytotoxics may be prescribed. The potential oral side-effects must be considered as well as the risk of haemorrhage.

Haemophilia and von Willebrand's disease

Dental care for this group poses major problems since neglect of oral hygiene can lead to dental emergencies which can be fatal unless carefully managed. Persistent bleeding following dental extractions may be the first sign of mild disease. Anaemia due to chronic blood loss may be a feature, and in von Willebrand's disease gingival bleeding is more common.

The risk of haemorrhage from dental extractions and of internal bleeding from routine intra-muscular injections of local anaesthetic requires carefully planned dental treatment. General anaesthesia poses the risk of accidental trauma during intubation. Treatment is always provided in

Medically Compromised Patients

consultation with the relevant haematology specialist. Pre-operative fibrinolytics or replacement of Factor VIII may be necessary, with detailed advice on post-operative care to reduce the risk of haemorrhage. The development of antibodies to Factor VIII makes haemorrhage more difficult to control and immunosuppressants may be prescribed.

Anxiety about the management problems associated with dental treatment may complicate the situation and delay the patient from seeking advice or treatment. The possibility of HIV carrier status from blood products may create further barriers. Dental extractions and crisis situations should be avoided; regular dental assessment, preventive advice and good oral hygiene are the keys to prevention and should be introduced at birth to reduce the life-threatening risks associated with congenital bleeding disorders.

Acquired bleeding disorders
These are commoner than congenital bleeding disorders. The main causes are summarised in *Table 13.6*.

Table 13.6 Causes of acquired bleeding disorders.

Anti-coagulant therapy
Aspirin
Indomethacin
Vitamin K deficiency
Malabsorption syndrome
Liver disease

Underlying disease, anaemia and drug therapy may complicate oral health and dental treatment. Adjustment of the patient's medication or antifibrinolytic therapy may be necessary in planned dental care. Oral preventive techniques are therefore essential to reduce the need for dental intervention.

13.5 Respiratory disorders

Respiratory disorders are well-known for their potential risk in general anaesthesia. The underlying cause and treatment may affect oral health, although the avoidance of general anaesthesia is the most important factor in dental management. Hospitalisation may be necessary for dental treatment under general anaesthesia.

Tuberculosis
In pulmonary tuberculosis, ulcers on the upper surface of the tongue may occur in a small proportion of patients (Chapter 14). General anaesthesia is

avoided and alcoholism and social deprivation may complicate oral health (Chapter 12). Rifampicin, which is prescribed as initial therapy may in rare cases cause oral lesions.

Cystic fibrosis

This disease is both hereditary and life-threatening, affecting the lungs and digestive system. Respiratory infections are common and treated with prolonged antibiotic therapy which may be sugar-based (Chapter 8). Malnutrition may be a consequence of impaired digestion with subsequent delay in growth and development. The development of diabetes mellitus and liver disease may complicate the condition. However, early diagnosis and careful management have improved life-expectancy.

Oral features may include enlargement of the salivary glands, defects in tooth surfaces (enamel hypoplasia) and delayed eruption of teeth. Tetracycline staining occurs with increasing rarity since tetracycline is no longer recommended for use during the period of tooth development (Chapter 8). Treatment with pancreatin may cause ulceration if the drug is retained in contact with oral tissues.

Despite dietary management to compensate for nutritional deficiency which may include a high cariogenic carbohydrate content, dental caries experience is generally lower.[9-11] A lower caries rate is thought to be due to long-term use of antibiotics. Studies demonstrate higher levels of calculus (tartar), which are thought to be related to the high calcium content of saliva in cystic fibrosis.[9]

General anaesthesia poses a major risk, and may be further complicated by diabetes and liver disease. Regular preventive dental care to remove calculus and avoid the need for general anaesthesia is essential.

Asthma

There are no oral features associated with asthma; however, long-term treatment with bronchodilators, systemic corticosteroids and steroid inhalers have potential oral side-effects (*Table 13.7*). Chronic mouth breathing may also contribute to a dry mouth.

Table 13.7 Oral side-effects of drugs used in treatment of asthma.

Inhalants	
Ketotifen	Dry mouth
Beclomethasone	Candidiasis
Budesonide	Candidiasis
Bronchodilators	
Ipratroprium bromide	Dry mouth
Systemic corticosteroids	Oral infection

13.6 Gastrointestinal disease

There are few oral features which significantly affect oral health that have not been covered in earlier sections.

Enamel erosion due to chronic or persistent acid regurgitation has been described in Chapters 2 and 12. Oral effects of anaemia secondary to malabsorption or haemorrhage are described earlier in this chapter. Diabetes mellitus may develop as a complication of pancreatic disease.

Glossitis, burning mouth and angular cheilitis (*Colour Plate* 24), together with recurrent ulcers, are early symptoms of coeliac disease. In Crohn's disease, swellings of lips or face and oral ulcers are reported oral symptoms, and ulcers may also occur in both Crohn's disease and ulcerative cholitis. Treatment with corticosteroids may complicate oral health.

Oral ulceration
This describes the commonest lesions affecting the oral soft tissues. Many are of no medical significance and may be due to localised trauma, e.g. from an ill-fitting denture. Recurrent ulcers occur in approximately 25% of the population and are associated with a range of factors such as diet, hormonal changes, vitamin deficiencies, and more. In a few rare cases, ulcers are a symptom of Behçet's syndrome, which may be due to immunodeficiency. Other causes have been described.

Ulcers normally take two weeks from the earliest oral changes to complete healing. As ulceration may occur as a symptom of more serious disease or secondary to medication, persistent or chronic ulceration merits referral for definitive diagnosis to exclude other conditions.

Dry mouth (xerostomia)
This is a symptom of reduced salivary secretion. It is referred to throughout the guide as being a high-risk factor for oral disease and discomfort. Causes are summarised in *Table 13.8* and oral care regimes described in Chapter 15.

Table 13.8 Causes of a dry mouth (xerostomia).

Infection
Drugs
Radiation
Dehydration

13.7 Liver disease

There are no significant oral features in relation to liver disease. However, anaemia and bleeding disorders may affect oral health and dental management. General anaesthesia is best avoided, unless managed by a specialist anaesthetist. The underlying cause of liver disease and its treatment must be considered.

13.8. Kidney disease

Oral features occur only in the less common renal disorders. Children with chronic renal failure exhibit delayed eruption, malpositioned teeth and enamel defects due to growth abnormalities. Signs and symptoms of anaemia and reduced salivary flow affect oral health. Bleeding and white patches due to keratin deposits (keratosis) may occur.

Corticosteroids and immunosuppressant therapy predispose to candidal infection. Transplant patients receiving long-term immunosuppressants are particularly at risk of oral infections. Cyclopsorin-induced gingival swellings may occur (*Colour Plate* 20). Antibiotic cover for certain dental procedures may be recommended.

Dental management may be complicated by steroids and immunosuppressants, anaemia, bleeding tendencies, anti-coagulant therapy, hypertension, and the underlying causes of liver disease. Steroid supplements and antibiotics may be required prior to dental treatment. General anaesthesia poses a severe management risk.

13.9 Diabetes

Dry mouth occurs in diabetes insipidus, which may also be secondary to head injury. Steroid therapy may complicate oral health. Diabetes mellitus has no specific oral features when well-controlled. If poorly controlled, oral health may be affected by dry mouth, delayed healing, susceptibility to oral infections and progressive periodontal disease (*Table 13.9*). Severe periodontal disease predisposes to tooth loss[12] and dental caries.[13] Certain anti-diabetic drugs such as chlorpropamide in rare cases cause white (lichenoid) patches.

Table 13.9 Oral complications in diabetes.

Dental caries	Dry mouth
Periodontal disease	Swollen salivary glands
Candidiasis	Glossitis

In diabetes mellitus, anxiety and stress associated with dental treatment may precipitate diabetic ketosis. Antibiotic cover for oral surgery may be required in poorly controlled cases. General anaesthesia may require specialist management.

13.10 Summary

While there are numerous rare conditions which may compromise oral health, the commonest and most significant non-malignant medical conditions and their treatment which affect oral health have been summarised. The avoidance of dental treatment under general anaesthesia is a priority for many of the conditions described. Techniques to maintain oral health, reduce plaque and eliminate extrinsic sugars are vital and should be implemented at the time of diagnosis. Regular dental attendance, for preventive advice and treatment which avoids crisis management, makes an important contribution to the maintenance of health.

13.11 References

1. Holbrook, W.P., Willey, R.F. and Shaw, T.R.D. (1981), Dental health in patients susceptible to infective endocarditis, *Br. Med. J.*, **283**, 371.
2. Urquhart, A.P. and Blinkhorn, A.S. (1990). The dental health of children with congenital cardiac disease, *Scottish Medical Journal*, **35**, 6, 166–168.
3. Pogrel, M.A. and Welsby, P.D. (1975). The dentist and prevention of infective endocarditis, *Br. Dent. J.*, **139**, 12–16.
4. Cawson, R.A. (1981). Infective endocarditis as a complication of dental treatment, *Br. Dent. J.*, **151**(12), 409–414.
5. Longman, L.P and Field, E.A. 1990. Prophylaxis of infective endocarditis – an update, *Dental Practice*, **28**(13), 1.
6. Scully, C. and Cawson, R.A. (1987). *Medical Problems in Dentistry*, 2nd ed. Wright, Bristol, p. 105.
7. Scully, C. and Cawson, R.A. (1987). *Medical Problems in Dentistry*, 2nd ed. Wright, Bristol, p. 107.
8. Van Dis, M.L and Langlais, R.P. (1986). The thalassemias: oral manifestations and complications, *Oral Surg.*, **62**, 229–233.
9. Kinirons, M.J. (1989). Dental health of patients suffering from cystic fibrosis in Northern Ireland, *Comm. Dent. Hlth.*, **6**, 113–120.
10. Jagels, A.E. and Sweeney, E.A. (1976). Oral health of patients with cystic fibrosis and their siblings, *Journal of Dental Research*, **55**, 991–996.
11. Blacharsh, C. (1977). Dental aspects of patients with cystic fibrosis: A preliminary clinical study, *Journal of the American Dental Association*, **95**, 106–110.
12. Albrecht, M., Benoczy, J. and Tamas, G. (1988). Dental and oral symptoms of diabetes mellitus, *Comm. Dent. Oral Epidemiol.*, **16**, 378–380.
13. Bacic, M. *et al.* (1989). Dental status in a group of adult diabetic patients, *Comm. Dent. Oral Epidemiol.*, **17**, 313–316.

14 Oral Infections and Related Conditions

14.1 Introduction
14.2 Candidiasis
14.3 Herpes virus infection
14.4 Epstein–Barr virus
14.5 Hepatitis virus
14.6 Human immunodeficiency virus (HIV)
14.7 Transmission of HIV
14.8 Oral conditions associated with HIV infections
14.9 Summary of HIV-related conditions
14.10 Oral health care for people with HIV infection
14.11 Cross infection control in oral care for people with HIV infection
14.12 Good practice guidelines for oral care
14.13 Summary
14.14 References

14.1 Introduction

The mouth contains a vast number of organisms, many of which are normally non-pathogenic but can become pathogenic when the immune defences are weakened. An example is *Candida albicans* which produces candidiasis, or thrush, often an indicator of underlying systemic disease.

Other oral infections may be primary infections; either relatively rarely seen, as in the case of tuberculosis, syphilis, and leprosy, or more common as with the herpes group of viruses.

Aside from the risk to the health status of the individual with an oral infection, there are also implications for infection of the health care professional involved in oral care. This is particularly relevant for viruses that may be identified in blood and saliva, and includes hepatitis viruses, the herpes group of viruses, and human immunodeficiency viruses (HIV).

Transmission between individual patients with the health care professional acting as a passive vector is of particular importance for older, frail or other compromised groups who are at risk from the spread of antibiotic-resistant bacteria, for example methicillin-resistant *Staphylococcus aureus* (MRSA). This bacteria is readily transmitted via hand, nasal or oral contact and can produce a life-threatening systemic infection.[1]

14.2 Candidiasis

Oral candidiasis (*Colour Plates* **22–25**) is a common fungal infection which is usually considered opportunistic with the presence of other factors, as shown in *Table 14.1*. It is the commonest infection in the mouth of individuals aged 70 and over, and the wearing of dentures strongly increases the candida oral population.[2]

Table 14.1 Factors which predispose towards oral candidiasis.

Age: very young or very old
Pregnancy
Local trauma due to ill-fitting dentures
Antibiotic therapy, particularly broad spectrum
Corticosteroids, both systemic and via inhalers
Malnutrition
Endocrine disorders
Malignancies including blood disorders
Immune defects including AIDS
Conditions producing dry mouth

Oral candidiasis is also one of the earliest signs of HIV infection and its presence in otherwise healthy individuals should be viewed with suspicion. Early referral is indicated as 50% of HIV-positive individuals can develop candidiasis[3].

The condition may show in four distinct presentations. In all cases smears of the area should be taken to confirm the diagnosis and detect drug-resistant strains.

Pseudomembranous candidiasis (thrush)

In this variant there are white meshes and patches on the mucous membranes of the cheek, tongue, or floor of the mouth. The pseudomembrane (literally 'false membrane') can be wiped off to leave a bleeding surface. The condition is treated with anti-fungal lozenges or suspension, e.g. amphotericin, nystatin and fluconazole.

Holistic Oral Care

Atrophic candidiasis

Atrophic candidiasis in a more chronic form is seen in 65% of denture wearers. The reddened, painless area is usually limited to the oral mucosa covered by the denture (*Colour Plate* 22). Treatment involves not wearing the denture at night and anti-fungal therapy. As the denture can act as a reservoir of infection, it should be thoroughly cleaned (Chapters 2 and 4).

The infection also presents as a reddened area on the palate and dorsum of the tongue, and is particularly seen after inhalation of steroids (*Colour Plate* 25). Treatment is the same as for pseudomembranous candidiasis. If it is possible to suspend the antibiotic or steroid therapy, this will hasten recovery.

Chronic hyperplastic candidiasis

This shows as white patches, nodules, or patches with red flicks in various sites around the mouth. The lesions should be excised and biopsied as there may be early signs of malignancy. Longer-term anti-fungal therapy may be indicated.

Candida associated angular cheilitis

This variant presents as chronic ulcers in the corners of the mouth (*Colour Plate* 24). Prior to the AIDS era it was usually confined to elderly denture wearers, who often had denture-related variants of candidiasis. In the denture wearer the condition may be caused by worn dentures making the person 'over closed', and new dentures with the correct vertical dimension may be needed. The ulcers may be secondarily infected from bacteria present on the skin and in the nostrils. The presence of angular cheilitis in younger groups should be investigated as a possible indicator of HIV infection.[4] Treatment consists of anti-fungal therapy.

14.3 Herpes virus infection

The commonest infections encountered in this group of viruses include herpes simplex I and II, varicella zoster and Epstein–Barr virus. These viruses produce a variety of infectious conditions and may also be associated with HIV infections and other underlying systemic conditions.

Primary herpetic gingivostomatitis

This oral infection is predominantly caused by the type I virus, although the type II virus, which used to be mainly restricted to genital lesions, is now often implicated.

Infection usually occurs in early childhood and presents in varying degrees of severity, ranging from mildly irritating vesicles in the mouth to much more severe oral ulceration, blood-encrusted lips and a raised temperature. The infection starts on the lips and mucous membranes as vesicles, which rapidly break down and ulcerate. The ulcers are then prone to becoming secondarily infected by oral bacteria. Healing is more rapid if the condition is treated early with systemic acyclovir, a specific anti-viral agent effective against herpes simplex. Once the ulcers are established, care of the mouth involves the use of antiseptic mouthwashes (chlorhexidine) and oral hygiene measures. The lesions tend to persist for 10–14 days and heal without scarring. They are very infectious, and there is a risk of spreading the infection to fingers, nose, eyes or genitals. Health workers involved in the care of patients with herpes simplex primary infections should practise a high standard of cross-infection control.[5]

Secondary herpes simplex infection

Nearly a third of patients who have suffered primary infection will subsequently suffer from secondary infections (*Colour Plate* 21) due to the reactivation of latent virus. The commonest site is on the lip, where it is commonly known as a 'cold sore', but it is occasionally seen in other sites in the mouth. A number of factors can provoke viral reactivation, including trauma, sunlight, and systemic upset. The lesion starts with a prickling sensation, followed by discrete vesicles which break down to form the distinctive crusted lesion that lasts 7–10 days. Treatment should be started early and consists of applications of topical acyclovir five times a day. The 'experienced' sufferer is usually aware of the early symptoms. Severe cases may require systemic acyclovir. The virus is present in saliva and mucosal membranes throughout the duration and special care should be taken by health workers to avoid infection. A minimal skin abrasion on non-gloved hands can lead to a painful intractable lesion, known as an 'herpetic whitlow', forming on the finger.[6]

Varicella zoster

This member of the herpes group also produces a primary infection and later reactivation of latent virus. The primary infection, chicken pox, is a common feature of childhood, and the lesions are occasionally seen as oral ulceration which may precede the skin rash. The secondary condition, shingles, is distributed in areas served by distinct nerves. The initial symptoms are pain followed by patches of ulcerations. Treatment consists of pain relief and systemic acyclovir therapy. The underlying condition should always be sought as a factor initiating the attack.

14.4 Epstein–Barr virus

Infection with the Epstein–Barr virus is responsible for infectious mononucleosis, transmitted in saliva. This condition, commonly known as 'glandular fever', consists of lymph node enlargement, fever and pharyngeal inflammation. Oral ulceration and small haemorraghic areas are seen in 30% of patients. The infection can range in severity from mild upset to a more serious condition affecting the liver and spleen. Oral care consists of limiting secondary infection with oral care and antiseptic mouthwash.

14.5 Hepatitis virus

This blood-borne infection has no oral lesions but remains important for the health professional involved in oral care because of the risk of transmission due to the presence of the virus in saliva. There are three variants, A, B and C with hepatitis B (HBV) being the most infective and very robust – which poses a challenge for cross infection control. The majority of patients infected with HBV are asymptomatic and may be unaware of their carrier status. The groups in *Table 14.2* are recognised as high-risk for HBV.

Table 14.2 High-risk groups for HBV infection

- Dental and other clinical staff, particularly where involved with drug dependency, haemodialysis, multiply-transfused patients.
- Laboratory staff in blood banks and pathology laboratories.
- Ethnic groups including immigrants.
- People living, or working, in institutions for those with learning disabilities.
- Those living, or working, in prisons or institutions with high-risk individuals, e.g. homosexuals, intravenous drug users.
- Immunocompromised patients.
- Long-term travellers from low to high prevalence areas.
- Partners and close relatives of the above.

In practice, it should be assumed that virtually every patient is a potential carrier, and the same high standard of cross infection control should be followed with all patients.

14.6 Human immunodeficiency virus (HIV)

Infection with HIV causes a disease which suppresses the immune system, leaves the individual susceptible to a wide variety of infections, and is linked to a group of otherwise rare tumours. The condition, acquired immune deficiency syndrome (AIDS), is unusual in that it is a form of immunodeficiency that is transmissible.

The increase in the number of cases throughout the 1980s has attracted worldwide attention and is being referred to as a global epidemic. The constantly changing outlook for the 1990s, regarding predicted cases and research into treatments or cures, is largely outside the remit of this book, but there is no doubt that the prevalence of HIV infection is very high. Current estimates of infected individuals are 1 in 40 individuals in Africa; 1 in 75 males, and 1 in 700 females in North America; and 1 in 200 males, and 1 in 1400 females in Western Europe.[7] A very high proportion (90%) of those individuals who are infected with HIV will develop AIDS, with the period between infection and the full-blown syndrome being constantly revised upwards.[7]

14.7 Transmission of HIV

HIV has been detected in blood, plasma, semen, saliva, tears and cerebrospinal fluid, with the main route of transmission being via sexual intercourse. There are a number of risk groups in society whose lifestyles are more likely to lead to transmission; these include people practising certain homosexual acts, and intravenous drug abusers. But with the huge increase in infection via heterosexual intercourse, it is not possible to identify all those individuals who are 'at risk'.

Although HIV can be detected in the saliva of infected individuals, it appears to be of a low infectivity compared to that found in other body fluids, but all health care workers should still maintain consistent cross infection control measures with all body fluid contacts.

14.8 Oral conditions associated with HIV infections

It is increasingly likely that the health care professional will be involved in providing care for people who are infected with HIV. Many will be symptom-free carriers and the first signs of AIDS developing may be seen in the mouth. There are also a number of conditions that are seen in HIV positive individuals that only involve the mouth. Currently, there are three groups of conditions associated with HIV infections (*Table 14.3*).[8]

Table 14.3 Conditions associated with HIV infection.

Group I Conditions strongly associated with HIV infection
Candidiasis
Hairy leukoplakia
HIV gingivitis
HIV periodontitis
Kaposi's sarcoma
Non-Hodgkin's lymphoma

Group II Conditions less commonly associated with HIV infection
Atypical ulceration (oropharynx)
Ideopathic thrombocytopenic purpura (blood platelet disorder)
Salivary gland diseases, including dry mouth and swelling of glands
Other viral infections including the herpes group and varicella

Group III Conditions possibly associated with HIV infection
Bacterial infections including actinomycosis, tuberculosis
Cat scratch disease
Fungal infections other than candidiasis
Facial palsy
Trigeminal neuralgia
Osteomyelitis
Sinusitis
Squamous cell carcinoma
Melanotic hyperpigmentation

Candidiasis
Because of the depressed immune system, it is vital that oral candidiasis (see 14.2) is treated to avoid its spread to the pharynx and oesophagus. Repeated and prolonged oral and systemic candidiasis is a common feature of AIDS.

Hairy leukoplakia
Hairy leukoplakia presents as white lesions on the margins of the tongue, which are not removable and do not respond to anti-fungal therapy. The tongue surface is sometimes corrugated in appearance. The lesion is an important early indicator of the progression from HIV positive status to AIDS.[8]

HIV gingivitis and HIV periodontitis
In an otherwise healthy clean mouth, the presence of a particularly severe form of gingivitis and/or periodontitis should be thoroughly investigated by the dentist, particularly if the condition does not respond to normal measures as described in Chapter 2.

Kaposi's sarcoma
This neoplasm was rare prior to the AIDS era, and was seen mainly in elderly Jewish males and people from Central Africa. It is now seen in 50% of AIDS sufferers, particularly in homosexual patients.[9] A diagnosis of Kaposi's sarcoma is accepted as defining a diagnosis of AIDS.[10] A typical site is the hard palate, and the lesion presents as a red or purple macule 1–2cm in diameter which is usually painless unless traumatised or ulcerated. The tumour is slow growing, does not metastasise, and treatment is usually palliative. Regression of the tumour has been observed in some patients receiving anti-retroviral treatments for the AIDS syndrome.[11]

Non-Hodgkin's lymphoma
This variety of lymphoma also presents as a reddish or purple swelling. It is more commonly found on the gingiva and the palatal mucosa.

14.9 Summary of HIV-related conditions

The list of conditions is wide and as research continues will probably expand, with some becoming more strongly associated as the number of HIV infections and cases of AIDS increases. The health care professional is clearly not intended to provide a detailed diagnosis of these conditions but the wider range listed does indicate the importance of an early referral to dental professionals when suspicions are aroused. As treatment regimes for AIDS develop, it appears vital that retroviral therapy is started early to control the condition. With many of the oral conditions acting as 'markers' for the conversion of HIV infection to AIDS, routine examination of the mouth by all health care professionals becomes more important.

14.10 Oral health care for people with HIV infection

Control and prevention of oral disease is important for people with HIV infection, as their deficient immune system will raise the severity and duration of any oral conditions. They may also be at risk due to the effects of retroviral therapy, chemotherapy or radiotherapy for lesions associated with AIDS. Treatment regimes may all produce xerostomia, which will further raise the risk of oral disease. *Table 14.4* shows the commoner oral complaints and their management.[12]

Holistic Oral Care

Table 14.4 Management of oral conditions.

Complaint	Management
Oral ulcers	Topical steroids or systemic steroids in severe cases
Candidiasis	Management of underlying xerostomia and anti-fungal therapy, particularly fluconazole. Chlorhexidine mouth rinses
Dental caries	Preventive care important; restriction of sugar intake. Fluoride supplements
Dental infections	Antimicrobial therapy, drainage
Gingival and periodontal infections	Vigorous oral hygiene procedures, chlorhexidine rinses
Herpes virus infection	Acyclovir therapy
Kaposi's sarcoma	Chemotherapy and/or radiotherapy
Pain	Careful investigation of cause and appropriate analgesics
Xerostomia	Saliva substitutes

14.11 Cross infection control in oral care for people with HIV infection

It is doubtful whether any other infective condition has aroused such strong emotions and fears throughout society. People with HIV infection have experienced intense stigma and fear from family, colleagues and society in general, almost reminiscent of leprosy or the bubonic plague. People with HIV infection have also experienced difficulties obtaining dental care once they have revealed their HIV status, with the stated reason for refusing treatment being insufficient cross infection control.[8] The risk of health workers becoming infected with HIV is low due to the relatively low infectivity of the virus compared to the hepatitis B virus. Although HIV can be demonstrated in the saliva of infected individuals, it is present in very much lower concentrations than in other body fluids[13] and the risk of transmission is more from direct innoculation with blood products. There are several basic principles of good cross infection control that should be practised by all health care workers involved in oral care. These principles are not specific to HIV and the same level of cross infection control should be practised for all patients.

14.12 Good practice guidelines for oral care

Vaccination against hepatitis B
Vaccination against Hepatitis B offers the best means of personal protection against the virus and will therefore benefit patients. It is recommended that all dental professionals should be vaccinated as well as other primary health care professionals involved in oral care where there is a risk of needle stick injury.

Medical history
Regular updating of medical history will alert to the possibility of being in a high-risk group.

Gloves/masks
Gloves should be routinely worn when health professionals are directly involved with mouth care. This includes carrying out or assisting with mouth care and the cleaning and handling of dentures.

Where there is a likelihood of creating a saliva/blood aerosol or spray, e.g. toothbrushing where there is a gum inflammation, then eye protection and a mask are recommended.

Disposal of waste
Disposable products should be used wherever possible and adequate provision made for the disposal of contaminated products, including sharps and needles, in safe containers.

Surface disinfectants
Effective surface disinfectants should be used routinely, and where possible disposal trays and covers.

Sterilisation
Effective sterilisation using boiling water is not adequate for HBV, and autoclaving at 134°C for a minimum of three minutes at 2.2 bar, or hot air at 160°C for at least 60 minutes, is required.[14]

14.13 Summary

Viral infections other than HIV can present in the mouth and pose a cross infection problem for health professionals. This is particularly relevant for the herpes group and hepatitis B virus. As many viral infections, including HIV, may be asymptommatic, all people should be treated as a potential risk. As HBV is the most infective, any cross infection guidelines should use control of transmission of this virus as the standard to achieve. However sensible, effective cross infection control can be carried out without it becoming a barrier to sensitive, patient-centred care.

14.14 References

1 Staat, R. H., Stewart, A. V. and Stewart, J. F. (1991). MRSA: an important consideration for geriatric dentistry practitioners. *Spec. Care Dent.*, **11** (5), 197–199.
2 Walker, D. M. (1991). Oral Disease. In: Pathy, M. S. J. (ed.) *Principles and Practice of Geriatric Medicine*, 2nd ed. Bristol, John Wiley, p. 385.
3 Lakshman, S. P. (1991). How to resolve oral candidiasis. *The Dentist*, July/August, 41–42.
4 Lakshman, S. P. (1990). Oral candidiasis: an old disease in new guises. *Dental Update*, Jan/Feb, 36–38.
5 Newton, T. (1991). Herpes remains as much of a problem as ever. *Dental Practice*, Sept. 7–8.
6 Lamey, P. J. and Lewis, M. A. O. (1989). Oral medicine in practice: viral infection. *Br. Dent. J.*, **166**, 269–274.
7 Challacombe, S. J. (1991). Oral research and dental treatment in HIV infection. *Br. Dent. J.*, **171**, 146–148.
8 Challacombe, S. J. (1991). Revised classification of HIV associated oral lesions. *Br. Dent. J.*, **170**, 305.
9 Ogden, G. R. and Chisholm, D. M. (1988). Orofacial manifestations of AIDS. *Dental Update* Dec., 420–423.
10 Speight, P. M., Zakrzewska, J. and Fletcher, C. D. M. (1991). Epitheliod angiomatosis as a first sign of HIV infection. *Br. Dent. J.*, **171** (11), 367–371.
11 Smith, D. and Croser, D. (1991). Oral manifestations of HIV disease. *Dental Practice*, Jan., 8–10.
12 Scully, C. and Luker, J. (1991). An ABC of oral health care in patients with HIV infection. *Br. Dent. J.*, **170** (4) 149–150.
13 Samaranayake, L. P. (1991) AIDS and dentistry – an update. *Dental Update*, July/August, 228–229.
14 British Dental Association (1991). Guide to blood borne viruses and the control of cross infection in dentistry. London, British Dental Association.

15 Malignant Disease and its Treatment

15. 1 Introduction
15. 2 Leukemia
15. 3 Oral malignancies and maxillofacial surgery
15. 4 Other malignancies
15. 5 Chemotherapy
15. 6 Radiotherapy
15. 7 Bone marrow transplantation
15. 8 Immunosuppression
15. 9 Oral care
15.10 Summary
15.11 References

15.1 Introduction

Advances in medicine have led to the development of new treatments for malignant disease. Early diagnosis and treatment improve life expectancy. Treatment regimes involve painful and distressing side-effects in addition to the emotional aspects of coping with cancer. Increased susceptibility to infection accompanies both disease and treatment. Furthermore, the mouth provides a pool of opportunistic infection which may lead to life-threatening systemic infection in individuals whose immunity system is already compromised by disease and/or treatment.

This chapter confines itself to the discussion of leukaemia and oral cancer, and also the oral aspects of treatment for malignant disease:

- Chemotherapy.
- Radiotherapy.
- Bone marrow transplantation.
- Immunosuppressive therapy.
- Surgery.

15.2 Leukaemia

Leukaemia is the collective term for a group of progressively malignant blood disorders characterised by large numbers of abnormal white blood cells. Increased susceptibility to infection is a direct result of failure in the defensive function of white cells. Anaemia and bleeding disorders are secondary to interference with normal bone marrow activity as white blood cells are produced at the expense of red blood cells and platelets. Leukaemias are classified according to the predominant blood cells affected and abnormality of cell structure. Acute leukaemias are differentiated from chronic leukaemias by the presence of immature or primitive white cells. Symptoms of leukaemia which affect oral health include:

- Increased susceptibility to infection.
- Bruising.
- Bleeding tendencies.
- Anorexia leading to poor nutritional status..

Acute lymphoblastic and myeloblastic leukaemia produce a similar clinical picture and without blood tests are indistinguishable. Oral symptoms are summarised in *Table 15.1*, although variations occur in the different types with gingival swelling commonest in myeloblastic leukaemia.

In over 10% of acute leukaemias, oral symptoms are the initial complaint[1]; painful and distressing symptoms may exacerbate the existing oral status. In the acute phase, normal oral hygiene techniques may need to be modified; nevertheless, every effort should be made to encourage and maintain oral hygiene: reduction of oral infection is a priority. Although chronic leukaemias are more common, they may convert to the acute type; the same principles of scrupulous oral hygiene apply.

During phases of acute oral infection, normal toothbrushing may be painful and potentially traumatic, providing the means for bacteria to enter the blood stream (bacteraemia) leading to systemic infection. Oral care may therefore be limited to mouthwashing with chlorhexidine gluconate (0.2%) at frequent and regular intervals to control plaque, together with appropriate

Table 15.1 Oral signs and symptoms of leukaemia.

Pale soft tissues
Gingival bleeding
Gingival swelling (red, soft or spongy)
Bruising (purpura)
Ulceration
Swollen tonsils
Swollen parotid salivary glands
Infections: candidiasis (*Colour Plates* 22–25)
 fungal infections
 herpes virus (*Colour Plate* 21)

Malignant Disease and its Treatment

antibiotic and anti-fungal therapy. Toothbrushing with a soft nylon brush and chlorhexidine gluconate gel should be carried out as soon as this can be tolerated, provided that it does not create a potential for bacteraemia. Toothbrushing and flossing should not be carried out when white cell and platelet counts are low (Chapter 9). It is important to consult the patient about the effectiveness of oral care techniques; this will provide guidance on the frequency and suitability.

Treatment with cytotoxics causes further oral complications (*Table 15.2*) with oral ulceration being a side-effect of most cytotoxics. Corticosteroids increase susceptibility to infection. Bone marrow transplants are increasingly used and offer an improved prognosis; however, the total body irradiation and chemotherapy which precede transplantation, in order to destroy all malignant cells, increase complications. Oral symptoms of irradiation are painful and are complicated by chemotherapy, immunosuppressive treatment and reaction to the transplant (*Table 15.3*). Oral symptoms of treatment and management of oral care are covered later in this chapter.

Table 15.2 Oral side-effects of cytotoxics.

Ulceration
Lip cracking
Gingival swelling
Bleeding
Salivary gland pain
Infections (particularly candidiasis)
Dry mouth (adriamycin)
Pigmentation (busulphan)

15.3 Oral malignancy and maxillofacial surgery

Early diagnosis of pre-malignant and malignant conditions improves prognosis for treatment (Chapter 1). The annual death rate from oral cancer in the UK is around 50%.[2] White areas of the mucous membranes or chronic ulceration should be investigated because of their potential for malignancy. Common sites for oral malignancy include the floor of the mouth, the border of the tongue and the lips, with squamous cell carcinoma being the most common type of oral carcinoma. Secondaries from malignancy in other sites may affect the jaws and rarer malignancies may occur. Although rare, lymphomas affect the salivary glands, in particular the minor salivary glands.

Diagnosis, assessment and treatment are interdisciplinary and the treatment regime selected is based upon a number of factors. Smaller localised lesions are generally treated with radiotherapy whereas larger, more extensive, lesions may be surgically removed with or without radiotherapy or chemotherapy. Acute oral mucositis, which may develop during or several weeks after radiation, involves the salivary glands. Oral side-effects may be minimised by the use of shields and splints, and fewer are experienced with the use of radiation implants. Side-effects include mucositis and xerostomia (dry mouth); preventive advice and maintenance of oral hygiene are a priority.

Surgery usually involves radical excision into healthy tissue beyond the margins of the cancerous lesion. Complex maxillofacial reconstruction and prostheses may be necessary to restore facial tissues and reduce disfigurement. Bone grafts may be used to restore the mandible. The patient will require sympathetic support to deal with the psychological aspects of disfigurement, as well as preventive oral care. Speech and swallowing may be impaired; and advice to ensure adequate nutrition may be needed. Multi-disciplinary support is essential for continuing post-operative care and maintenance of oral health. An organisation set up to assist sufferers cope with the social handicap of facial disfigurement provides comfort and support in rehabilitation and social integration.[3]

15.4 Other malignancies

It is beyond the scope of this guide to discuss this vast and complex area. Secondaries from breast, lung, thyroid, kidney, stomach and prostate cancer may occur in the mouth – the jaws being the most frequent site. Systemic effects of malignancy may also present in the mouth. Treatments for malignancy have the potential to seriously affect oral health. The oral side-effects of chemotherapy, radiotherapy and immunosuppressants have already been described. Maintenance of oral health, comfort and function is a priority in these at-risk groups.

15.5 Chemotherapy

Oral side-effects of cytotoxics may exacerbate oral symptoms (*Table 15.2*). A high standard of oral hygiene is essential to prevent and reduce the severity of oral complications and to prevent the potential for systemic infection secondary to oral infection. Caries and periodontal disease due to poor oral hygiene and xerostomia increase the risk of systemic infection. Chemical plaque control is essential, as is gentle but efficient manual plaque control when white cell and platelet counts are raised. Saliva substitutes may help to relieve dry mouth and denture hygiene should be scrupulous. Continued attention to oral hygiene after chemotherapy and in remission is essential. Topical fluoride may be introduced when the individual can tolerate it.

Malignant Disease and its Treatment

Oral assessment and any extractions or oral surgery should be carried out before chemotherapy in liaison with the oncology consultant. Dental care which is provided in consultation with the oncology team may be necessary prior to chemotherapy to reduce the risk of oral infection.

15.6 Radiotherapy

Radiation affecting the head and neck contributes to a number of oral complications (*Table 15.3*). The degree of oral involvement depends upon the type, dose and duration of treatment and the tissues irradiated. Generalised stomatitis may affect all soft tissues. Reduced salivary gland function which causes xerostomia may take many months to return to normal function, if at all. Patients need advice in coping with these symptoms, since they may not be continuously hospitalised and mayreceive treatment as an out-patient.

Mucositis, characterised by red inflamed soft tissues which eventually slough off, is extremely painful and can substantially hinder completion of cancer therapy.[4] Soreness and dysphagia may develop after radiotherapy and eventually subside. Dentures are removed or worn sparingly and always removed at night.[4]

The symptoms of xerostomia have been described earlier in this guide. Saliva may become thick, ropey and viscous shortly after radiotherapy. Xerostomia increases the risk of caries, periodontal disease, oral and salivary gland infections. Both xerostomia and damage to taste buds contribute to loss of taste.

Table 15.3 Oral complications of radiotherapy to head and neck.

Mucositis:	redness
	sloughing
	discomfort
Xerostomia:	caries
	periodontal disease
	candidiasis
	salivary gland inflammation/infection
	dysphagia
Loss of taste:	xerostomia
	damage to taste buds
Radiation caries	
Hypersensitive teeth	
Osteoradionecrosis and osteomyelitis	
Trismus	
Dental defects	

Dietary changes to cope with painful oral conditions and nutritional requirements may increase the risk of caries. This may be complicated by radiation caries caused by direct damage to the developing tooth structure in younger patients[5] and reduction in salivary flow and reduced salivary pH.[4] Cavities on the smooth surfaces of teeth and encircling the crowns at the gingival margins are characteristic of radiation caries (*Colour Plate* **11**). Topical fluoride to prevent radiation caries and chemical plaque control (chlorhexidine gluconate) is essential. Saliva substitutes provide some relief, although preventive measures may be painful during phases of acute mucositis.

Radiation damage to bone increases the risk of developing osteoradionecrosis, therefore healing is delayed. This is the rationale for extractions to be carried out prior to radiotherapy because of the risk of osteomyelitis following radiation. Good oral hygiene reduces the risk of complications during and after radiation treatment.

15.7 Bone marrow transplantation

Bone marrow transplantation is a therapeutic technique used for the treatment of a number of blood dyscrasias and malignant conditions which do not resolve with chemotherapy (*Table 15.4*).[6]

Table 15.4 Conditions that are treated with bone marrow transplant.

Acute leukaemia	Aplastic anaemia
Chronic leukaemia	Fanconi's anaemia
Preleukaemic states	Thalassaemia
Lymphoma	Sickle cell anaemia
Multiple myeloma	Selected solid tumours
Neuroblastoma	

Bone marrow tissue is obtained from three sources (*Table 15.5*). Graft versus host disease (GVHD) is a complication in allogeneic transplants and leukopenia in syngeneic transplants. The effect of chemotherapy and radiation on bone marrow and the presence of residual malignant cells are major disadvantages in autologous transplants.

Chemotherapy and total body irradiation are carried out approximately 5–10 days pre-transplant for all types of bone marrow transplantation. These are performed in isolation, as the patient is even more vulnerable to infection during this period. Prognosis is best when transplant is carried out in remission. Complications arise due to a number of factors (*Table 15.6*).

Malignant Disease and its Treatment

Table 15.5 Sources of bone marrow.

- Allogeneic: healthy tissue from a compatible sibling.
- Syngeneic: healthy tissue from an identical twin.
- Autologous: tissue from the patient's own bone marrow.

Table 15.6 Complications of bone marrow transplantation.

- Poor nutrition
- Debilitation due to cytotoxics
- Impaired healing
- Systemic bacterial infection
- Latent viral infections
- Impaired systemic defence
- Immunosuppression

Oral complications of bone marrow transplantation are exacerbated by radiotherapy and chemotherapy (*Table 15.7*). In graft versus host disease, healthy bone marrow cells develop an immunological response to host tissues; this is further complicated by the host's immunosuppression from chemotherapy and radiotherapy. Immunosuppressive therapy is necessary post-transplant to suppress GVHD (*Table 15.7*). Cyclosporin causes less mucositis than methotrexate since it is less toxic to bone marrow. Oral complications are worse in acute GVHD although chronic GVHD may develop from the acute form and occur 2–3 weeks post-transplant.

Table 15.7 Oral effect of graft versus host disease

Desquamation	Mucosal erythema
Ulceration	Mucosal atrophy
Chelitis	Non-specific pain
Lichenoid patches	Xerostomia
Keratoses	

Additional complications due to myelosuppression and immunosuppression from chemotherapy and radiotherapy lead to opportunistic infections and mucosal atrophy. Xerostomia and lowered salivary pH increase the risk of caries. Patients with exposed roots are reported to develop extensive root caries.[7,8] Xerostomia which persists requires lifetime care with saliva substitutes; topical fluorides are essential for the dentate to increase enamel resistance to caries.

15.8 Immunosuppression

Immunosuppressive treatment has complex implications and side-effects. Cytotoxics used to prevent rejection of grafts or transplants have an immunosuppressive effect by interfering with normal cell division. Drugs which have direct and indirect immunosuppressive effects are summarised in *Table 15.8*.

Increased susceptibility to infection is a side-effect of both types of drugs. Cyclosporin is not toxic to bone marrow and has less severe side-effects than other cytotoxics, although gingival hyperplasia (swelling) may occur.

Table 15.8 Immunosuppression.

Non-cytotoxic drugs:	Corticosteroids	
	Cyclosporin (*Colour Plate* 20)	
Cytotoxic drugs:	Azothiaprine	Lomustine
	Busulphan	Melphalan
	Carmustine	Mercaptopurine
	Chlorambucil	Methotrexate
	Cyclophosphamide	Mitobronital
	Cytarabine	Mustine
	Estramustine	Thioguanine
	Fluorouracil	Thiotepa
	Ifosfamide	Treosulfan

15.9 Oral care

Oral side-effects of malignant disease and treatment are complex and may be life-threatening. The objectives of oral care are:

- Relief of oral pain, distress and discomfort.
- Prevention and treatment of oral infection.
- Prevention of caries, periodontal disease and soft tissue pathology.
- Maintenance of oral health and function.

Practical aspects of oral care from the nursing perspective are summarised by Daeffler[9]:

- Keep oral mucosa clean, soft, moist and intact
- Keep lips clean, soft, moist and intact
- Remove debris and plaque without damaging mucosa
- Eliminate oral pain and discomfort.

Malignant Disease and its Treatment

Oral care techniques described in Chapter 2 provide the basic knowledge required. The type of oral intervention required will depend upon:

- Stage of illness or disease.
- Type and intensity of treatment.
- Previous oral health status.

Planned dental treatment and prevention at diagnosis are important. Close liaison between the oncology and dental teams will ensure that the most effective and appropriate techniques are used. It is important to include subjective assessment on the effect and frequency of oral hygiene regimes. A summary of oral hygiene regimes follows; however, it must be stressed that if white cell and platelet counts are low, toothbrushing and flossing are discontinued in favour of chemical plaque control.

Reduction in the risk of opportunistic infection is a priority. A fall in the white cell and platelet counts signals the need to discontinue normal oral hygiene techniques.[10] Foam mouth sticks are recommended during the period of isolation in bone marrow transplantation.[10] Gentle swabbing using a finger wrapped in gauze is useful for the edentulous patient. However, the most important tool for mouthcare is a small soft toothbrush; soaking in 1% sodium hypochlorite or chlorhexidine solution helps to keep the brush soft. Replacement before the filaments bend and cause trauma is essential.

Chlorhexidine gluconate, which is bacteriostatic in low concentrations and bactericidal in high concentrations, has been demonstrated to be effective both in the control of bacterial plaque[11] and in the management of mucositis and candidal infection.[12,13] It is recommended for plaque control when toothbrushing is suspended and in conjunction with normal oral hygiene techniques when white cell and platelet counts are raised.

Denture hygiene should be scrupulous and dentures stored in 1% hypochlorite solution or a similar proprietary brand to reduce candidal infection; it is frequently recommended that dentures are removed during treatment. Professional and self-applied topical fluoride reduce the risk of caries, in particular radiation caries. Saliva substitutes provide relief for xerostomia. Regular individual oral assessment is essential to ensure that the correct oral hygiene techniques are being used in relation to the oral, general and haematological status.

Oral care regimes based on Scully's recommendations[14] are summarised in *Tables 15.9–15.11*.

Table 15.9 Oral hygiene and oro-dental care at diagnosis and prior to radiotherapy and chemotherapy

- Identification of appropriate oral hygiene techniques.
- Training in mechanical plaque control for teeth, soft tissues and appliances, with guidance and supervision of a dental hygienist.
- Chlorhexidine gluconate mouthwash (0. 2%).
- Professional scaling and prophylaxis may be provided if the white cell and platelet count is adequate.
- Relief of dental pain and elimination of potential sources of oral infection.
- Elimination of potential causes of oral irritation, e.g. sharp teeth, orthodontic appliances, rough or ill-fitting dentures.
- Relief of oral ulceration: Warm saline mouthwash.
  Lignocaine hydrochloride 2% in a viscous gel.
  Benzydamine hydrochloride 0.25%.
  Frequency is decided by the prescriber and monitored.
- Topical fluoride for dentate patients.

Table 15.10 Oral care during radiotherapy and chemotherapy

- Regular oral assessment
- Maintenance of appropriate oral hygiene techniques
- Removal of oral appliances
- Relief of xerostomia: Saliva substitutes
  Frequent sips of water
  Ice chips
  Atomised water sprays
  High moisture foods
  Avoidance of spicy foods
  Fluids with meals
- Mucositis: Chlorhexidine gluconate mouthwash (0.2%)
  Warm normal saline mouthwash
- Ulceration: as above
- Oral infections: Antifungal/antiviral therapy
  Chlorhexidine gluconate mouthwash (0.2%)
- Periodontal disease: Mechanical plaque control
  Chlorhexidine gluconate M. W. (0.2%)
  Chlorhexidine gluconate gel (1%)
- Dental caries: Dietary control of sugars
  Topical fluoride
- Dental hypersensitivity: Topical fluoride
- Trismus: Regular jaw exercises
- Lips: Clean with gauze and normal saline
  Moisten with lanolin-based lubricant
- Angular cheilitis: Clean with gauze and normal saline
  Antifungal/antiviral ointment

Malignant Disease and its Treatment

Table 15.11 Oral post care radiotherapy, chemotherapy and BMT transplantation.

- Maintenance of oral hygiene.
- Chemical plaque control (Chlorhexidine gluconate).
- Dietary control of sugars (dentate).
- Topical fluoride (dentate).
- Saliva substitutes for chronic xerostomia.
- Regular oro-dental assessment.

15.10 Summary

Oral care for cancer patients is a topic discussed with increasing frequency in nursing journals.[15-19] However, the rationale for many interventions does not appear to have a clear scientific basis.[20] There is obviously a need to carry out more research into the current methods for prevention and alleviation of oral complications.

Within the interdisciplinary team, the oncology nurse has a particularly important role to play in patient education and support. Day to day mouthcare is in the province of nursing rather than medicine[19]. Regular oral assessment, and ensuring the availability of the most appropriate tools and materials, ensuring that appropriate oral hygiene techniques are carried out and assessed at regular intervals, form the basis of good nursing intervention[21] (Chapters 6 and 9). Prevention and palliation of oral complications enhance the patient's comfort, improve the quality of life and reduce the risk of serious systemic infection.

15.11 References

1. Scully, C. and Cawson, R. A. (1987). Leukaemia and other malignant disease. In: *Medical Problems in Dentistry*, Bristol, Wright, p. 119.
2. Office of Population Censuses and Surveys. *Mortality Statistics: Cause. Reviews of the Registrar General on deaths by cause, sex and age in England and Wales, 1985.* London: HMSO, 1987, Series DH2 No. 12.
3. *Let's Face It*, Christine Piff, 10 Wood End, Crowthorne, Berkshire, RG11 6DQ.
4. Rothwell, B. R. (1987). Prevention and treatment of the orofacial complications of radiotherapy, *Journ. Am. Dent. Ass.*, **114**, 316–322.
5. Gorlin, R. J. and Mishkin, L. H. (1963). Severe irradiation during odontogenesis, *Oral Surg.*, **16**, 35–38.
6. Appelbaum, F. R. (1988). Marrow transplantation for haematological malignancies: a brief review of current status and future prospects, *Sem. Hemetol.*, **25**, suppl. 3, 16–22.

7. Heidt, P. J. (1988). Management of bacterial and fungal infections in bone marrow transplant recipients and other granulocytopenic patients, *Canc. Detect. Prevent.*, **12**, 609–619.
8. Seto, B. G. *et al.* (1985). Oral mucositis in patients undergoing bone marrow transplantation, *Oral Surg.*, **60**, 493–497.
9. Daeffler, R. (1980). Oral hygiene measures for patients with cancer, *Cancer Nursing*, **3**, 6, 427–432.
10. Maxymiw, W. G. and Wood, R. E. (1989). The role of dentistry in patients undergoing bone marrow transplantation, *Br. Dent. J.*, **167**, 229–234.
11. Addy, M. (1986). Chlorhexidine compared with other locally delivered antimicrobials: a short review, *J. Clin. Periodontol.*, **13**, 957–964.
12. Ferretti, G. A. *et al.* (1987). Therapeutic use of chlorhexidine in bone marrow transplant patients: case studies, *Oral Surg.*, **63**, 6, 683–687.
13. Ferretti, G. A. *et al.* (1987). Chlorhexidine for prophylaxis against oral infections and associated complications in patients receiving bone marrow transplants, *JADA*, **114**, 461–467.
14. Scully, C. (1985). Patients with malignant disease. In: *Hospital Dental Surgeon's Guide*, BDJ, Latimer Press, Plymouth, pp. 84–87.
15. Crosby, C. (1989). Method in mouthcare, *Nursing Times*, **85**, 35, 38–41.
16. Watson, R. (1989). Care of the mouth, *Nursing*, **3**, 44, 20–24.
17. Williams, L. T. and O'Dwyer, J. L. (1983). Guidelines for oral hygiene, denture care, and nutrition in patients with oral complications. In: Peterson, D. E. and Sonis, S. T. (ed.) *Oral Complications of Cancer Chemotherapy*, Martinus Nijhoff, London, pp. 151–168.
18. Allbright, A. (1984). Oral care for the cancer chemotherapy patient, *Nursing Times*, **80**, 21, 40–42.
19. Campbell, S. (1987). Mouthcare in cancer patients, *Nursing Times*, **83**, 29, 59–60.
20. Richardson, A. (1987). A process standard for oral care, *Nursing Times*, **83**, 32, 38–40.
21. Jenkins, D. A. (1989). Oral care in the ICU: an important nursing role, *Nursing Standard*, **4**, 7, 24–28.

16 Oral Care of the Dysphagic, Dependent and Terminally Ill

16.1 Introduction
16.2 Normal swallowing
16.3 Dysphagia (impaired swallow)
16.4 Oral care for dependent or dysphagic patients
16.5 Oral hygiene equipment and materials
16.6 Oral care in terminal illness
16.7 Summary
16.8 References

16.1 Introduction

In providing or supervising oral care for dependent or unconscious patients, it is essential to ensure that the airway is protected. Oral care for individuals with dysphagia (impaired swallow) requires careful management. An understanding of the swallowing process is necessary before the most appropriate and safe method of oral care can be selected.

Dysphagia combined with impaired mental function may limit the standard of oral care which can be provided. Nevertheless, oral care regimes can be adapted to individual problems and make a significant contribution to the individual's oral comfort and sense of well-being.

16.2 Normal swallowing

Swallowing can be divided into three phases: oral, pharyngeal and oesophageal. The oral phase is mainly voluntary; it can be initiated or arrested at will. The involuntary phase, once initiated, triggers the pharyngeal phase. Both pharyngeal and oesophageal phases are involuntary. Mastication involves complex sensory and motor function. Salivary secretion, stimulated by the presence of food, acts as a lubricant to facilitate mastication and swallowing. When mastication is complete, the tongue, aided by oral musculature, collects food, rolls it into a bolus and pushes it posteriorly. Liquids are swallowed immediately and succulent foods very quickly.

Swallowing may be a function of how rapidly foods stimulate salivary flow. During this phase, lips are closed and the soft palate is lowered, protecting the airway. When the tongue propels food into the pharynx, the swallow reflex, which takes approximately one second, is triggered. Once swallowing is initiated, involuntary pharyngeal and oesophageal stages continue. Breathing is temporarily arrested during the pharyngeal stage and the airway protected until the bolus reaches the oesophagus.

16.3 Dysphagia (impaired swallow)

Dysphagia may occur due to failure of one or all of the stages described and has a number of possible causes; organic causes are summarised in *Table 16.1* and psychogenic causes in Chapter 12. It may occur as a complication of radical surgery for treatment of carcinoma or due to fibrosis following radiation therapy (Chapter 15).

Primary concerns are the maintenance of nutrition and protection of the airway. If oral nutrition is inadequate, non-oral feeding is implemented alone or as a supplement to oral feeding. The risk of aspiration increases if there is:

- Impairment or delay in the involuntary phase of swallowing.
- Impairment of the laryngeal protective mechanism.
- Loss of sensation in the area.
- Absence of cough reflex.

Problems confined to the oral voluntary stage may affect the type and quantity of nutrition. Liquids are more difficult to manage, while moist

Table 16.1 Causes of dysphagia

- Xerostomia
- Inflammatory lesions in the throat
- Foreign bodies
- Paterson–Kelly syndrome
- Pharyngeal pouches
- Benign swellings
- Carcinoma
- Scleroderma
- External pressure
- Neurological and neuromuscular disorders: Achalasia
　　　　　　　　　　　　　　　　　　　　　Syringobulbia
　　　　　　　　　　　　　　　　　　　　　Cerebrovascular accident (stroke)
　　　　　　　　　　　　　　　　　　　　　Cerebrovascular disease
　　　　　　　　　　　　　　　　　　　　　Motor neurone disease
　　　　　　　　　　　　　　　　　　　　　Guillain–Barré syndrome
　　　　　　　　　　　　　　　　　　　　　Poliomyelitis
　　　　　　　　　　　　　　　　　　　　　Diphtheria
　　　　　　　　　　　　　　　　　　　　　Cerebellar disease
　　　　　　　　　　　　　　　　　　　　　Myopathies: Myasthenia gravis
　　　　　　　　　　　　　　　　　　　　　Muscular dystrophies
　　　　　　　　　　　　　　　　　　　　　Dermatomyositis

Dysphagic, Dependent and Terminally Ill

puréed meals facilitate swallowing. Problems with the pharyngeal stage can cause choking, coughing and aspiration; non-oral feeding is usually implemented. Surgical intervention is necessary for problems with the oesophageal stage if reflux occurs. The presence of a tracheostomy tube increases the risk of aspiration.

Other factors which affect swallowing are summarised in *Table 16.2*. The infantile swallow is characterised by a tongue thrust. Primitive oral reflexes may develop as a result of cortical deficit and cranial nerve involvement; tongue thrust and bite reflex pose problems for oral care. It is necessary to do an oral assessment, identify the type and degree of dysphagia, and whether or not there is a cough reflex, before planning oral care techniques.

Table 16.2 Other factors which affect swallowing.

Ability to form lip seal	Underactive and hyperactive gag reflex
Loss of sensation	Delayed oral swallow
Reduced awareness of food residues	Primitive oral reflexes

Interdisciplinary assessment, involving speech therapy, physiotherapy and dietetics, provides the necessary information for the management of oral care. Desensitisation techniques to promote oromuscular activity may be recommended by the speech therapist.

Drooling is generally a symptom of dysphagia rather than of excessive salivation. It may be due to any of the factors given in *Table 16.2*, as well as to tongue thrust, neuromuscular inco-ordination, structural abnormalities, intra-oral irritation or posture. Social unacceptability, skin rashes, and the need for special clothing are factors which have lead to the development of methods for management of drooling. Surgical redirection of the salivary gland ducts, removal of salivary glands and other more complex techniques have been reported.[1] Anticholinergic drugs are rarely used because of their lack of specificity for salivary glands. Behaviour modification is described for those with learning difficulties with some success.[2]

Palatal-training appliances attached to teeth or dentures are used with varying success in the management of both drooling and speech problems; a reduction in drooling and speech problems has been attributed to use of the devices in stroke patients.[3] Success is reported in some patients with cerebral palsy, although there is no method of assessing whether the situation would have improved without therapy.[1] Palatal-training appliances are reported in the management of speech problems.[4,5] Further research is necessary to identify criteria for successful outcome in the use of these devices. However, their continued use is justified by the dental profession.[1]

In the stroke patient, prostheses may be designed, or dentures modified, to support sagging musculature by eliminating the sulcus. This increases denture stability and food is prevented from accumulating on the affected side.[3] A prosthesis which plumps the lower lip is reported for the management of drooling in a case of amyotrophic lateral sclerosis.[6]

Oral health may be at risk due a number of factors (*Table 16.3*). Calculus (*Colour Plates* **5, 6**) is reported to form significantly faster in tube-fed individuals, and therefore plaque removal is a priority.[7] Orodental assessment may offer alternative management strategies, as well as identifying oral hygiene needs in dysphagia.

Table 16.3 Factors affecting oral health.

- Lack of oromuscular activity.
- Poor lip posture.
- Mouth-breathing.
- Food accumulation due to sensory loss or paralysis.
- Dietary changes.
- Xerostomia (dry mouth).

16.4 Oral care for dependent or dysphagic patients

Posture is important in assisting swallowing; if possible, the individual should be seated upright with feet firmly on the ground. Tilting the head backwards hinders swallowing, and a slight increase in flexion is recommended.[8] If the patient is bedridden, the head should be tilted forward; and if reclining, the patient's head should be tilted to one side to assist drainage. With unilateral facial paralysis, the head should be tilted away from the affected side.

Whenever possible, oral care should be given from behind the patient (*Figure 4.3*). In people with cerebral palsy, the loss of neck support and movement of the head from the midline will trigger the tonic labyrinthine and asymmetrical tonic neck reflexes, respectively. These reflexes can be minimised by supporting and cradling the head and neck from behind the patient. It may be easier to provide oral care with the patient in the prone position.

Oral assessment (Chapter 6) identifies the type of oral care suitable for the individual patient. This assessment should be done by the nursing staff on admission and evaluated regularly to review oral status and oral hygiene needs. Nurses are recommended to routinely inspect the mouth with a pen torch and spatula prior to providing oral care.[9] Subjective assessment of oral comfort and satisfaction should be included.

Recommendations for practical oral care adapted from previously reported nursing guidance are summarised in *Table 16.4*.[9,10]

Table 16.4 Summary of oral care for the dependent patient

- Prepare appropriate oral hygiene materials.
- Place the patient in the sitting or semifowler's position to protect the airway.
- Protect clothing.
- Wear gloves.
- Remove dentures or other removable appliances.

Dentate patient
- If necessary, insert a mouth prop to gain access.
- Floss interproximal surfaces of teeth, taking care not to traumatise gingivae.
- Brush all surfaces using fluoride toothpaste or chlorhexidine gel.
- Rinse or aspirate to remove saliva and toothpaste.

Dentate and edentulous patients
- Gently retract cheeks and brush inside surfaces with soft gentle strokes.
- Using gauze to hold the tongue, gently pull the tongue forward and brush surface gently from rear to front.
- Gently brush palate.
- Towel or swab mouth if toothbrushing is not possible.
- Aspirate throughout procedures if airway is at risk.
- Lubricate lips as necessary.

Dentures and removable appliances
- Brush vigorously with unperfumed household soap.
- Pay particular attention to clasps.
- Rinse well in cold water.
- Saliva substitute may be required before replacing the denture in the mouth.

Intubated patients
- Reposition tube frequently to prevent lip soreness.
- Ensure tube is secure before proceeding with oral care.
- Proceed with oral care as appropriate.

16.5 Oral hygiene equipment and materials

These are summarised in Chapter 9. In severe dysphagia, aspiration is essential to protect the airway and to ensure that toothpaste is not left in the oral cavity; an aspirating toothbrush may be useful (Chapter 9).

Chlorhexidine gel does not foam and provides chemical plaque control (Chapter 9). Gauze swabs soaked in chlorhexidine gel or mouthwash provide an alternative when toothbrushing is impossible. Foam sticks may also be used in this way, but are less effective than conventional oral hygiene techniques[11-13]; they may be hazardous if the foam end becomes detached.

For post-surgical care, the type and frequency of post-operative oral care is under the direction of the maxillofacial team. In postsurgical care or in maxillary fixation, chlorhexidine mouthwash is essential provided there is no risk of aspiration. Straws can be used to deliver mouthwash. Oral irrigation devices with aspiration are beneficial, and can also be used to deliver mouthwashes (Chapter 9).

Holistic Oral Care

The mouth and fixation should be cleaned gently with a soft toothbrush; chlorhexidine gel may be preferable to toothpaste. Chlorhexidine spray is another method of achieving chemical plaque control. Dried blood and blood clots may be removed with sodium bicarbonate mouthwash.[14]

Dentures should be removed for cleaning and at night. The mucosa and tongue may be cleaned by gentle brushing with a small soft toothbrush or by towelling and swabbing. Saliva substitutes may be necessary for the xerostomic subject (Chapter 9). Dry and crusted lips may be bathed with saline and lubricated with KY or a lanolin-based cream. Vaseline should not be used as it has been implicated in aspiration pneumonia.[15] Dietary adjustment should take account of the risk of caries from extrinsic sugars for the dentate patient.

16.6 Oral care in terminal illness

The priority in terminal illness is to provide comfort and relief of painful or distressing symptoms in prolonging active life and in the terminal stages of life. Subjective assessment is even more important and oral hygiene techniques should be modified according to reported symptom relief.

Constant reassessment of the oral status and evaluation of techniques and materials are the key to effective palliative oral care. The patient's right to refuse oral care should be respected.

Oral health in the terminally ill has received little attention. Seventy per cent of deaths in palliative care programmes are due to malignant disease.[16] Oral symptoms, which include soreness, ulceration, glossitis, candidal infection and xerostomia, have a serious impact on quality of life.[17] A recent study in the UK on subjective oral symptoms in hospice patients confirms the high percentage with oral symptoms (Table 16.5).[18] Fifty per cent had some degree of gingival inflammation, and other oral pathologies were noted. Of the 75% who wore dentures, 71% had difficulty with their dentures, while 60% wore their dentures overnight. Many dentures were old and unsatisfactory due to weight loss, and yet denture relines provided at the bedside can offer a rapid solution to ill-fitting dentures. High levels of oral candidal infection, diagnosed in 70% of the patient sample, have been confirmed by other studies of terminal illness.[19-21] Furthermore, pain relief with opiate derivatives may exacerbate xerostomia.[22]

Table 16.5 Reported oral symptoms in hospice patients.

Symptom	Percentage of patients
Taste	26%
Dysphagia	37%
Soreness	42%
Dryness	58%

The effects on the oral cavity of malignant disease and its treatment have been discussed in Chapter 15. Since deaths reported in hospice care are mainly due to malignant disease[16], and oral symptoms are commonly reported, there is clearly a need to include the dental team in an holistic approach to terminal care. Both Berkey[23] and Lapeer[24] argue the case for incorporating dentistry into the palliative care team, so that the orodental needs of the dying may be managed more effectively.

Oral care regimes are based on the relief and improvement of symptoms. Although oral candidiasis does not appear to correlate directly with oral symptoms, topical treatment with nystatin or miconazole is recommended when candidiasis and loss of taste occur together[19]. Detailed regimes depend on oral and subjective assessment; techniques and materials are covered in this and other chapters. *Table 16.6* summarises the principles of palliative oral hygiene.

Table 16.6 Principles of palliative oral hygiene.

Removal of plaque and food debris
Denture hygiene and use
Relief of xerostomia
Relief of other reported symptoms

16.7 Summary

This chapter summarises the principles of oral care for those who are mainly dependent on others for oral hygiene. The contents are of particular importance for the professional nurse and should be read with Section 1 and Chapters 9 and 15.

Although there are clear medical imperatives for effective oral care to minimise the effects of oral and dental disease, an additional objective is the reduction of discomfort and improved quality of life for people undergoing painful and unpleasant treatment regimes. To be able to converse, eat and drink comfortably are basic human needs that are even more important for the person with a debilitating or terminal condition.

If there is one connecting theme running through Section 3, it is the need for close collaboration between all members of the health care team, including the dental team. Although it is the primary health care professional who will be helping the patient with day-to-day maintenance of oral health, it is the authors' contention that this task can be supported and augmented by close links with the dental team.

16.8 References

1. Oliver, R.G. (1987). Theoretical aspects and clinical experience with the palatal-training appliance for saliva control in persons with cerebral palsy. *Spec. Care in Dent.*, Nov.–Dec., 271–274.
2. McCracken, A. (1978). Drool control and tongue thrust therapy for the mentally retarded. *Am. J. Occup. Ther.*, **32**, 79–85.
3. Selley, W.G. (1977). Dental help for stroke patients. *Br. Dent. J.*, **143**(120), 409–412.
4. Enderby, P., Hathorn, I.S. and Servant, S. (1984). The use of intraoral appliances in the management of acquired velopharyngeal disorders. *Br. Dent. J.*, **157**, 157–159.
5. Thompson, R.P.J., Ferguson, J.W. and Barton, M. (1985). The role of removable orthodontic appliances in the investigation and management of patients with hypernasal speech. *Br. J. Orthod.*, **12**, 70–77.
6. Moulding, M.B. and Koroluk, L.D. An intraoral prosthesis to control drooling in a patient with amyotrophic lateral sclerosis. *Spec. Care in Dent.*, **11**(5), 200–202.
7. Dicks, J.L. and Banning, J.S. (1991). Evaluation of calculus accumulation in tube-fed, mentally handicapped patients: the effects of oral hygiene status. *Spec. Care in Dent.*, **11**(3), 104–106.
8. Langley, J. (1987). Management. In: Garvill, D.C. (ed.) *Working with Swallowing Disorders*. Bicester, Winslow Press, p. 54.
9. Mouthcare. In: Pritchard, A.P. and David, J.A. *The Royal Marsden Hospital Manual of Clinical Nursing Procedures*. 2nd ed. London, Harper and Row, p. 238.
10. Williams, L.T. and O'Dwyer, J.L. (1983). Guidelines for oral hygiene, denture care, and nutrition in patients with oral complications. In: Peterson, D.E. and Sonis, S.T. *Complications of Cancer Chemotherapy*. London, Martinus Nijhoff, p. 163.
11. De Walt, E. (1975). Effect of timed oral hygiene measures on oral mucosa in a group of elderly subjects. *Nr. Research*, **24**, 104–108.
12. Shepherd, G. Page, C. and Sammon, P. (1987). Oral hygiene. *Nursing Times*, **83**(19), 25–27.
13. Harris, M.D. (1980). Tools for mouthcare. *Nursing Times*, **76**(8), 340–342.
14. Scully, C.M. (1985). Definitive management of maxillofacial injuries. In: British Dental Association. *Hospital Dental Surgeon's Guide*. Plymouth, Latimer Press, p. 210.
15. Prakash, U.B. and Rosenow, E.C. (1990). Pulmonary complications from ophthalmic preparations. *Mayo Clin. Proc., Lul.*, **65**(4), 521–529.
16. Buckingham, R.W. and Lupu, D. (1982). A comparative study of hospice services in the United States. *Am. J. Public Health*, **72**, 455–461.
17. Gordon, S.R., Berkey, D.B. and Call, R.L. (1985). Dental needs among hospice patients in Colorado: a pilot study. *Gerodontics*, **1**, 125–129.
18. Aldred, M.J. et al. (1991). Oral health in the terminally ill: a cross-sectional pilot survey. *Spec. Care in Dent.*, **11**(2), 59–62.
19. Finlay, I.G. (1986). Oral symptoms and *Candida* in the terminally ill. *Br. Med. J.*, **292**, 592–593.
20. Pople, J. and Oliver, D. (1986). Oral thrush in hospice patients. *Nursing Times*, **82**, 34–35.
21. Clarke, J.M.G., Wilson, J.A., von Haacke, N.P. and Milne, L.J.R. (1987). Oral candidosis in terminal illness. *Health Bull.*, **45**, 268–271.
22. White, I.D., Hoskins, P.J., Hanks, G. and Bliss, J.M. (1989). Morphine and dryness of the mouth. *Br. Med. J.*, **298**, 1222–1223.
23. Berkey, D.B., Ofstehage, J.C., Crane, C.A. and Malley, K.J. (1987). Is there a role for dental professionals within hospice programs? *J. Palliative Care*, **3**, 35–37.
24. Lapeer, G.L. (1990). The dentist as a member of the palliative care team. *J. Can. Dent. Assoc.*, **19**, 56, 3, 205–207.

Section 4

Oral Health Promotion: Approaches and Practices

Introduction to Section 4

This section comprises two chapters on oral health promotion. It is aimed at the primary health worker whose role includes promoting, improving and maintaining their clients' oral health. Of course, in general, all primary health workers are involved, as the promotion of health is one of their most important roles. But it is the experience of many in the dental team that oral and dental health are often low down on the list, if on it at all! This may be because dental disease is rarely life-threatening, not forgetting that oral cancers have a similar mortality rate to cervical cancers.[1] Nevertheless, dental disease causes much suffering, and the treatment of dental caries and periodontal disease is a significant drain on the resources of health care systems. Ill-fitting dentures and the associated pathology are a handicapping condition that restricts normal function and reduces the quality of life.[2]

Methods of preventing oral disease are quite simple and have been reiterated throughout this book: restrict sugar intake, practise effective oral hygiene, use fluoride and maintain regular dental attendance. The difficulty is for everyone to have access to these processes and to be able to put them into practice. It is our contention that one of the problems is that dental and oral health have been outside the mainstream of health promotion for too long. There are many possible reasons for this. The long existence of a speciality dedicated to the treatment of oral disease has inevitably led to a 'ring-fencing' of the whole area of dental and oral health. This argument was raised in Chapter 3, in discussing a preventive strategy for child dental health, but it applies in equally valid measure to other client groups. The lack of dental and oral disease training in the curricula of most primary health professionals is a significant barrier which we hope this guide will redress! As a result, the health professional is forced to rely on personal oral health skills and knowledge. Many of us who are trained in a speciality inevitably find ourselves being the 'well-informed individual' when dealing with health issues outside our subject, and we find ourselves relying on information gathered from working within a multi-disciplinary team. The same dilemmas face the voluntary and informal carer.

There are already a wealth of texts and research into health and health behaviour, although not many specifically on oral health. This section will examine some of the main aspects of oral health and related behaviour to identify how oral health fits into general health-related behaviour. An understanding of these behaviour patterns is as much health promotion as any extolling of the preventive dental messages.

The lack of access to specialised knowledge might seem disadvantageous, but it is just because of this that the primary health care professional has a vital role in oral health promotion. People consult other health professionals and knowledgeable lay carers about dental health concerns precisely because they are not intimately linked with any actual treatment. Fear and anxiety of dental treatment form a well-established barrier to seeking dental care.

The second chapter of this section describes some of the practical strategies that primary health professionals can use to deliver oral health education and health promotion programmes. Chapter 18 aims to show in a practical sense how the primary health care professional and carer can be involved in oral health promotion. The preceding Chapter 17 describes an appropriate model and approach, and describes opportunities for health promotion throughout life. The main client areas of the individual, the family and the community are used as a base for interventions. These groups will inevitably overlap because people belong to different groups in a community; a child belongs to a family, and is a school student and a member of a peer group. A common theme running through the three groups is the role of the oral health promoter with others in the primary health care team, whether formal or informal. Thus the podiatrist working with the older adult can also help promote oral health by being alert to an individual seeking advice on an oral problem. This could be for example a persistent mouth ulcer with sinister implications.

What we are advocating is not merely an appendage or complementary to health promotion undertaken by the dental team, but oral health promotion carried out as an integral part of primary health care. It is about reaching groups not in contact with dental services.

The core knowledge required by an effective oral health promoter is contained in Section 1 of this guide. This can be backed up in the UK by the publication, *The Scientific Basis of Dental Health Education*.[3]

There are no real differences in the techniques used to promote oral health from those dealing with other dental issues. The primary health care worker is already using skills of counselling, teaching, demonstrating, empowering, lobbying and networking. Extensive skills in oral diagnosis and treatment are not required provided access to professional dental services is obtainable. In most northern, industrialised countries this should not present a problem. However, in southern, developing countries the primary health care professional may have to provide more clinical oral services. Readers who find themselves in this situation should consult Murray Dickson's source book, *Where there is no dentist*.[4]

References

1. Johnson, N.W. and Warnakulasariya, K.A.A.S. (1991). Oral cancer: is it more common than cervical? *Br. Dent. J.*, **170**, 5, 170–171.
2. Smith, J and Sheiham, A (1979). How dental conditions handicap the elderly. Comm. Dent. *Oral Epidemiol.* **7** 305:10
3. Health Education Authority. (1989). *The Scientific Basis of Dental Health Education*. 3rd ed. London, HEA.
4. Dickson, M. (1983). *Where there is no dentist*. The Hesperian Foundation, USA.

17 Approaches to Oral Health Promotion

17.1 Introduction
17.2 Health promotion and primary health care
17.3 Perceptions of health and oral health
17.4 Health and illness behaviour
17.5 Illness behaviour
17.6 Health behaviour
17.7 Maximising oral health potential
17.8 Oral health status
17.9 Oral disability and oral handicap
17.10 Chain of oral disability
17.11 Oral health promotion
17.12 A model of health promotion
17.13 Oral health promotion activities
17.14 Summary
17.15 References

17.1 Introduction

This chapter examines aspects of health and health status and how oral health is integrated into these approaches. The way in which illness affects behaviour and the ability to function is examined, first in a general sense and then from an oral perspective. However, this analysis is carried out for more than a descriptive purpose: it is intended to maximise the effectiveness of preventive interventions.

I7.2 Health promotion and primary health care

The main approaches to health care in the last decade have been shaped by the Primary Health Care Approach (PHCA).[1] This refocused the approach to illness and disease from a purely curative model and included a preventive and rehabilitative aspect based on health promotion. However, the resultant

Approaches to Oral Health Promotion

plethora of new terms and health-planning vocabulary has also given rise to some confusion to health workers who, rightly, have always seen themselves as striving towards a preventive approach. For further reading on the role of the PHCA in dental care see *The Practice of Primary Dental Care*.[2]

Whatever the terminology or model used, health workers are not just in the business of *providing health care* for people, they are also involved with helping people do it for *themselves*.

The Ottawa Charter for health promotion[3] states:

Health promotion is the process of enabling people to increase control over, and to improve, their health. To reach a stage of complete physical, mental and social well being an individual or group must be able to identify and realise aspirations, to satisfy needs and to change or cope with the environment.

How and where health workers get involved in the health promotion process will vary. Certainly, health promotion is not purely the domain of health care organisations, it involves governments, both local and national, and other major decision-makers. The opposite of this is that, although at first glance health promotion is all about 'macro' decision-making and environmental change, there is an important component of 'micro' changes for individuals. These processes will be based on health education to promote selfcare and to maximise their health potential. The success of this will depend on the skills of the health worker in their inter-reactions in many cases.

As this guide is primarily orientated towards health workers outside of the dental team, the preceding paragraphs may appear self-evident. The issues relating to re-orientating other members of the health team are already well underway. They are being addressed in Project 2000, and the first standard for Health Visiting practice[4] states:

Health visiting actions are positively directed towards health promotion and foster the client's ability to maximise his/her health potential.

17.3 Perceptions of health and oral health

Health for many people is a useful social product, a tool to help them with day-to-day living. It is something that is taken for granted until there is a change in health status.

As part of the obsession of western, scientific-based society, there are many attempts to dissect and classify what is meant by 'good health'. One of the more useful is the classification into physical, mental, emotional, social, spiritual and societal health.[5] Linked to this is the view of health in a 'holistic' fashion, where all these components are seen together and it is the relationship and balance between the various sectors that produce 'good health'. In theory there should not be any real need for deep philosophical contemplations about what is meant by 'good oral health'.

The problem arises with the dichotomy between health professionals' views of health and the views of the general public on what constitutes good health. If not as individuals, then as a group, the health care profession is still firmly grounded in the medical model of health. Indeed, many health professionals instinctively reach for the support of the medical model with its specialised knowledge of disease systems to provide the sort of cause and effect arguments used to back up much health education. But we know that for many people health is not seen in this context. Good oral health is something that is expressed often in purely functional terms: the mouth that works, that is pain-free and has an acceptable appearance. Oral and dental diseases are very widespread[6] but it is only when they impinge on any of the three criteria that they become an issue. The 'common sense' view that people adopt to oral health with a purely functional base goes some way to explaining why oral health is often left out of mainstream health contemplations. Could it be that most health professionals, outside of the specialised dental area, view oral health in the same way as members of the public, albeit well-informed members?

Oral and dental diseases remain a major health issue and it is clear that, although there have been large in-roads, the traditional curative medical approach has failed to achieve the goals of oral health for all. It is vital that oral health promotion measures are included in the mainstream of health promotion, for it is in the mixture of public health measures, environmental and social changes, and measures to educate and influence social norms that the route to good oral health lies.

17.4 Health and illness behaviour

Although these two types of behaviour are inter-linked, there are some differences. The stages that people go through when they perceive themselves to be 'ill' tend to be more linear and progress through a number of clear stages. This may be due to the fact that, as they are suffering from symptoms, they do actually have a definite organic problem. The stages they experience in health-related behaviour are more complex and will tend to interact and reflect more the person's values and beliefs and those of their family, the community and society. However, at key positions in both sets of behaviour timely interjections by primary health care professionals can be seen to be health-promoting.

17.5 Illness behaviour

Many people use the dental services mainly for the treatment and alleviation of symptoms, despite urging by the dental profession to visit for a more preventively orientated purpose.[7] Before they actually get to the stage of visiting the dentist, they will have passed through a series of stages, including: recognising that there is a problem, and coming to a decision about what to do about it – which may include consulting someone first. This has been described as an 'illness career'[8], and the primary health care professional has an important role in the individual's transition through these stages and the eventual outcome. At any stage, the individual or their parent/guardian may seek advice from a non-dental health worker, or the symptoms may appear as a disorder in another part of the body, e.g. earache, headache, loss of appetite.

Worldwide studies[9] suggest that there is actually a huge unmet demand for dental care as opposed to the actual expressed need. This has been popularly described as the 'iceberg'[10] of unmet need. The symptoms range from soreness of soft tissues in the mouth, bad breath, broken teeth to actual pain. It is how people deal with these symptoms that is the critical factor. The first step is deciding that the symptoms constitute a sufficient problem to disrupt normal life and to be abnormal. At this early stage there is a clear indication that the person should have access to correct information as to what is and what is not abnormal. This will partly reflect the cultural values of the community and society, for example that it is normal for dentures to cause pain when eating or that it is normal for children to develop cavities in their teeth that are painful. Perhaps one of the commonest ignored symptoms which the dental profession would regard as abnormal is the bleeding of gums when brushing. This is a clear indication that chronic marginal gingivitis is present.[11] Once the symptoms have been identified, they can either be suppressed or ignored, or the person may decide to seek some advice. This may be from family or friends, the so-called 'lay referral'[12] system, or a non-dental health worker. At this point self-treatment of the condition may be suggested by whoever is consulted, in order to avoid a dental visit. This could be semi-medicalised, i.e. non-prescribed analgesics or other home remedies or traditional treatments. Unfortunately, although self-treatment at this stage may reduce the symptoms, failure to treat the cause will only prolong the condition. The final link in the career is to seek a dental visit.

It is the complexity of people's behaviour and the influence of others around them in their families and the community that act as a filter, so that most dental symptoms never reach the stage of a visit to the dentist. The primary health care professional is more intimately involved with the community and is at a pivotal position to advise on which symptoms will require treatment.

17.6 Health behaviour

Although avoiding symptoms and illness behaviour are important aspects of health behaviour, there are other factors which will motivate people regarding their health. There is a balance between the costs and the benefits of taking health actions. For example, controlling the intake and frequency of sugar consumption to avoid dental caries, or visiting the dentist every six months compared to non-restriction and only visiting when having symptoms like toothache. People need to feel that the balance is on the side of 'benefit'. This can be difficult if the benefits are not immediately apparent. An example would be trying to convince an adolescent of the need for good oral hygiene to avoid the effects of periodontal disease in later life. The short-term benefits in this case would be a more attractive appearance and fresher breath. If however, the individual feels that they are 'at risk' and susceptible to the condition, they are more likely to take a health action, provided it appears to be the right one for them. This type of health-related behaviour has been described in the Health Beliefs Model.[13] However, the complexity of human behaviour has introduced other factors as to what might trigger people into action and most models are unable to provide the complete picture.

The decision is not always as clearcut as costs versus benefits. Sometimes decisions are made even though the individual knows there are costs but these are judged to be relatively minor compared to other factors. A simple example would be the dilemma of a parent with a crying child who chooses a sugar-containing drink because that will pacify the child and not disturb others asleep in the home. In this case there is a health compromise as a clearcut healthy choice is not available.

The type of health behaviour adopted will also be affected by the beliefs, values and habits that the individual has acquired. This process of social learning, *socialisation*[14], is an important process in the development of an individual's oral health behaviour. During the primary socialisation phase, which takes place in the home during the pre-school years, the basic patterns of diet and oral care are laid down. An early introduction to sweet foods, particularly as a token of affection or reward, will become a life-long habit. Early patterns of social grooming, including mouth care, are also established at this stage, along with the types of coping behaviour for dealing with symptoms of oral disease. Later on, as the child grows, the influence of the peer group becomes more important in the selection of diet. The decision to consume sugar-containing snacks is particularly open to influence by peer groups.[15] These influences can be used equally for health-promoting behaviour despite the undoubted expertise of the sugar industry in promoting the consumption of its snacks and drinks by the use of role models and other peer influences.

17.7 Maximising oral health potential

The now famous World Health Organisation definition of health[16] as:

a state of complete physical, mental, and social well-being, rather than solely as an absence of disease

Approaches to Oral Health Promotion

has often been criticised as being Utopian and practically impossible to attain. As the prevalence of oral disease is still very widespread and oral symptoms are suffered by over 20% of the population at any one time[17], it is quite plain that the goal *is* unattainable for most of the population, even with the recent decline in oral disease. It is therefore more applicable for the goal of oral health promotion to be maximising the potential for oral health and minimising oral disability and the resulting oral handicap.

Chapter 1 has addressed the way in which general disability can contribute to an oral disability, but oral conditions themselves are disabling which can lead to social handicap.

17.8 Oral health status

As a starting point for maximising oral health, it is necessary to ascertain the current health status, in order to assess meaningfully any improvement. This is not as clear as first examination would suggest. There already exist many indices, as used by dental epidemiologists, to assess individual and community health needs, but most measure present or past disease levels as opposed to oral health. They can very accurately predict the treatment needs but have limitations in assessing health status.[18]

Effective indicators for oral health status are still in development[19], but most proposed include some aspect of not just disease levels and levels of symptoms but also the personal and social consequences of the disease. This type of socio-dental indicator of oral disease would need to be able to look at disease, disability, discomfort and dissatisfaction. To a certain extent the dentist would make that type of assessment during a complete examination, diagnosis and treatment plan, but it is rarely made explicit and quantified.

A similar comparison would be to the sickness impact profile[20], which examines the effects of disease on 12 major areas of daily living (*Table 17.1*).

Table 17.1 Sickness impact profile categories.[20]

Physical	Ambulation
	Mobility
	Body care and movement
	Sleep and rest
	Eating
Psycho-social	Social interaction
	Alertness behaviour
	Emotional behaviour
	Communication
Social roles	Work
	Home management
	Recreation and pastimes

Reproduced with permission of J.B. Lippincott Co., Philadelphia, USA.

Some of the more explicit categories are already in existence and are yielding information concerning the impact of oral disease. An example from each of the major categories demonstrates the considerable impact on the individual and society.

Social roles
Studies of days of work lost due to dental disease reveal that 7.1 million days of work are lost each year in the USA.[21] Cushing[22] found that 26% of employed adults in England had suffered dental pain and 50% had had oral discomfort in the previous year. There are clear social costs to oral disease which have effects on national economies.

Physical
Eating is an obvious important function of the oral cavity, and the enjoyment of food and eating is a quality-of-life issue. Problems of eating are more likely in the denture wearer as the chewing efficiency of a denture is only 12% that of natural teeth[23], and a third of denture wearers experience some difficulty chewing[24]. Even though it is difficult to ascertain whether this has an effect on nutritional intake, it will certainly restrict the diet to that which can be more easily handled by dentures. It is not only denture wearers who experience difficulties with eating. Cushing found that 20% of her sample of 16–60 year olds experienced problems eating. Many of these problems were caused by hypersensitivity of teeth to hot and cold foods.

Psychosocial
A restricted diet will also affect the normal social roles of eating. Embarrassment about poor oral functioning can also drive people to eat alone. General dissatisfaction with appearance is a source of embarrassment which alienates people from normal social activities. The appearance of teeth and mouth are important in the self-esteem of the individual, an attractive smile is a valued trait in physical attraction.

17.9 Oral disability and oral handicap

Oral disease produces a range of limitations in normal function both at a personal oral level and socially, i.e. an oral disability. This individual disability may mean that they cannot conform to their expected role or position in society through being unable to take part in normal activities. Society or social groups can turn the disability into a handicap which will disadvantage them further. This is directly linked to quality of life and opportunities for that person. Oral handicap is a term that is difficult to define and to measure because it involves so many dimensions, including loss of opportunity, deprivation and dissatisfaction. Research undertaken on the subject of the handicap caused by facial appearance has shown its affect on children's school performance[25], and has also shown that people with congenital facial deformities may have their marital-life chances affected.[26]

Smith and Sheiham[27] in their study of how dental conditions handicap the elderly, noted how embarrassment and social discomfort caused by ill-fitting dentures deterred them from eating in public and made them self-conscious about their appearance and about speaking. To demonstrate that this is a rectifiable condition, Baxter[28] showed how the provision of new dentures improved confidence in social eating and decreased reticence about eating in public. Interestingly, although their nutritional status didn't alter, people felt an improvement in well-being.

17.10 Chain of oral disability

Oral disease and subsequent effects are linked in a simple model:

Oral disease ⟶ Impairment ⟶ Functional limitation ⟶ Oral disability ⟶ Handicap

The primary health care professional can interfere with this chain in the primary stages by recognising the oral disease and therefore reducing the impairment, and at later stages by tackling the functional limitation and reducing the oral disability. Although this may sound rather theoretical and jargon-laden, the actions are much more practical.

17.11 Oral health promotion

In the introduction, we stated that this section was concerned with the practicalities of oral health promotion. So far, this chapter has examined how oral health fits in with general health and illness and, of course, there is little special about oral health issues in comparison with other areas. For the reader to appreciate this point we would regard as one of our major aims accomplished! Hopefully, we can apply the same rationale to oral health promotion: that is, to integrate it more fully into general health promotion models and methods.

Holistic Oral Care

17.12 A model of health promotion

Most people involved in health over the last decade cannot fail to have been affected by the rise of the health promotion movement, in the way that they view how they deliver their service. The philosophy, terms and methods arose from the 'Health for All 2000' declaration.[29] Because it was a global declaration involving co-operation between countries, workers at the ground level can be forgiven for failing to see its relevance to them in their daily work. The term 'health promotion' has become an umbrella term to describe a range of activities. These include health education, prevention, legal, fiscal and environmental methods which have a common aim to promote positive health, maximise health potential and prevent ill-health. There are a wealth of texts which examine models, methods and techniques of health promotion in all its component parts (see References at the end of this section). One of the most easily understood models of health promotion is that shown in *Figure 17.1*.[30]

The three spheres of activity give rise to seven domains of action which can equally be applied to oral health promotion.

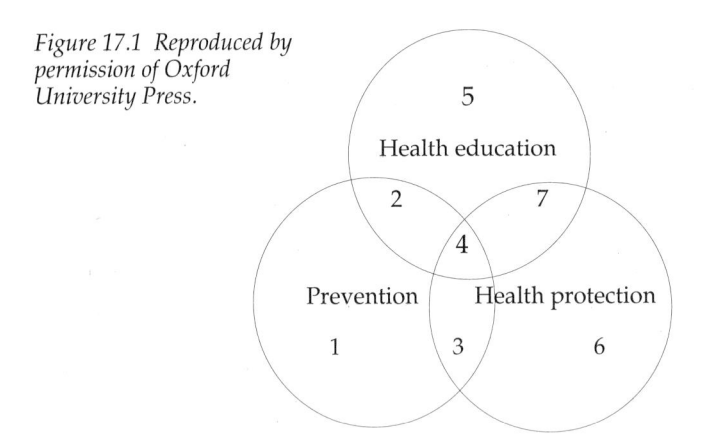

Figure 17.1 Reproduced by permission of Oxford University Press.

A Venn diagram of three overlapping circles labelled Health education (5), Prevention (1), and Health protection (6), with overlap regions numbered 2, 4, 7, and 3.

17.13 Oral health promotion activities

Using the seven domains described by Downie, Fyfe & Tannahill[31] we will describe seven activity areas within which primary health care professionals and carers may be involved. A degree of overlap is caused by inability of any model to capture the full range of appropriate methods. It is safe to say that, as there are still considerable sections of the dental professions who do not appreciate the value of a full integration of oral health promotion into the wider field, that task itself can be included as

Approaches to Oral Health Promotion

an health education activity. The practicalities of the 'training of trainers' as a health promotion method are considered in Chapter 18.

Preventive services
Preventive services frequently involve the direct activities of health professionals. Although many of the preventive methods are in the field of the dental profession, fissure sealants, prophylactic professional cleaning, and fluoride applications, other activities involve other members of the health care team. These may include denture cleaning and oral care, identification of high-risk individuals and screening, in addition to the screening activities of the dental team.

Preventive health education
These educational activities are aimed to promote a more orally healthy lifestyle and will include health education concerning diet, oral practices and use of dental services. As sizable proportions of the population only use dental services for treatment of symptoms and not for preventive reasons, other members of the health care team will have access to the groups that are, arguably, most at risk in society. A less disease-based example of a healthy oral lifestyle influence, is the promotion of gum shields and oral protection for contact sports.

Preventive health protection
These methods are concerned with encouraging an environment which is healthier, and where healthy choices are easier choices.[32] With regard to oral health, the single most effective way of improving health protection would be fluoridation of water supplies. Although individual health workers cannot initiate this themselves, support during any consultative process to implement fluoridation is vital. It is important to redress the balance from anti-fluoridationist objections and general societal and community apathy.

Aside from fluoridation, supporting moves to limit the advertising of sugar products aimed at children, supporting moves for more effective food labelling at national levels and promoting the formulation of healthy eating policies at schools and work places are all oral health protection activities. Of course, these may be construed as 'political' and not necessarily the role of the primary health worker, but recognising that these health promotion methods are political also recognises that health in itself has the same 'political' aspects.

Health education for preventive health protection
Activities in this domain involve methods that mobilise individuals to press for, and implement, healthy changes via a process of health education. An example could be alerting parents of children at a play group of

the oral health risks in the snacks and drinks provided and encouraging them to draw up a healthy food policy, and on a national level mobilising the considerable force of 'consumers' to alert them to health risks in sugar-containing infant drinks. As with any action which involves individuals lobbying and pressing for change, there are often considerable barriers to overcome. Probably the major one is persuading individuals that they can have an influence. The recent rise in consumerism related to health risks in food has amply demonstrated that influence does exist even when there is little co-ordination or planning.

Positive health education
This activity is described as aimed at influencing behaviour on positive health grounds and helping individuals, groups and communities to develop these attributes.[33] This is unlikely to be primarily focused on oral health but is a good example of where oral health can be incorporated into 'holistic' health considerations. There are certainly opportunities for encouraging positive oral health and the benefits of a healthy mouth. With much earlier dental health education being focused on avoiding dental disease, highlighting positive oral health is a progression to ways in which people themselves view health in a non-medical style.

The fatalism that many people display about the inevitability of their contracting dental disease may be countered by positive health education. This type of health education is aimed at the stereotypical view of the older person with dentures. Although expectations about the life of dentitions are rising the concept of 'teeth for life' still is not widespread.

Positive health protection
This area is closely linked with preventive health protection. As the concept of positive oral health is still a new and unfamiliar one, the activities of promoting policies and promoting healthy environments can be placed under both groups. An oral example could be the replacement of sugar-containing snacks in schools not just with high-fat crisps, but with more positively healthy snacks such as fruit. The exercise then becomes more than mere damage limitation – replacing one health risk with another – it promotes positive general health.

Health education aimed at positive health protection
This, similarly, has considerable overlap with the other domains of health protection and will encompass awareness raising, and raising expectations. This will not just be with individuals but also with policy makers and those with influence, including colleagues in the primary health care team!

17.14 Summary

- We have demonstrated that health promotion is an integral part of primary health care.
- We have examined some aspects of health and illness to highlight how oral health can be integrated.
- We have looked at how oral disease can produce social handicap in itself.
- We have described how oral health promotion should be integrated into health promotion activities.

17.15 References

1. WHO (1978). *Alma Ata 1978: Primary Health Care. Report of the International Conference on Primary Health Care*, Alma Ata, USSR. 6–12 September 1978. Geneva, World Health Organisation (Health For All Series No.1).
2. Jacob, M.J. and Plamping, D. (1989). *The Practice of Primary Dental Care*. Butterworth.
3. Ottawa Charter (1986). *An International Conference on Health Promotion*. World Health Organisation.
4. Royal College of Nursing (1989). *Standards of Care for Health Visitors*. RCN Scutari.
5. Ewles, L. and Simnett, I. (1985). *Promoting Health: a practical guide to health education*. Wiley, pp. 3–18.
6. Health Education Authority (1989). *The most common disease in the world?* DH19, London, HEA.
7. Gift, H.C. (1984). Utilisation of professional dental services. In: Cohen, L.K. and Byrant, P.S. *1970 Social Sciences and Dentistry: A critical biography*, Vol. 2, Quintessence. London.
8. McKinlay, J.B. (1971). The concept of patient career as a heuristic device for making medical sociology relevant to medical students. *Soc. Sci. Med.*, **5**, 441–460.
9. WHO (1976). Planning and evaluation of public dental health services, Technical Report Services 589, International Collaborative Study of Dental Manpower Systems. Interim Report, WHO, Geneva.
10. Last, J. (1963). The clinical iceberg: completing the clinical picture in general practice. *The Lancet*, **2**, 28–31.
11. Smith, D.G. (1990). Primary prevention of periodontal disease. *Dent. Update*, Aug., **17**, 6, 226–233.
12. Freidson, E. (1960). Client control and medical practice. *Am. J. Sociol.*, **65**, 374–382.
13. Haefner, D.P. (1974). The Health Belief Model and preventive dental behaviour. *Health Education Monogr.*, **2**, 420–432.
14. Blinkhorn, A.S. (1978). Influence of social norms on toothbrushing behaviour of pre-school children. *Community Dent. Oral Epidem.*, **6**, 222–226.

15. Rise, J. and Holund, U. (1990). Prediction of sugar behaviour. *Community Dental Health,* **7,** 267–272.
16. WHO (1946). Constitution, WHO, New York.
17. WHO (1985). *Oral Health Care Systems: An international collaborative study.* Quintessence, London.
18. Locker, D. (1989). *An Introduction to Behavioural Science and Dentistry.,* Tavistock/ Routledge, p. 76.
19. Locker, D. (1989). *An Introduction to Behavioural Science and Dentistry.,* Tavistock/ Routledge, p. 79.
20. Bergner, M. and Bobbitt, B. (1981). The sickness impact profile: development and final revision of a health status measure. *Medical Care,* **19** 787–805. In: Locker, D. (1989). *An Introduction to Behavioural Science and Dentistry.* Tavistock/ Routledge.
21. Locker, D. (1989). *An Introduction to Behavioural Science and Dentistry.,* Tavistock/ Routledge, p. 89.
22. Cushing, A., Sheiham, A. and Maizels, J. (1986). Developing socio-dental indicators – the social impact of dental disease. *Community Dental Health,* **3,** 3–17.
23. Locker, D. (1989). *An Introduction to Behavioural Science and Dentistry.,* Tavistock/ Routledge, p. 94.
24. Cushing, A., Sheiham, A. and Maizels, J. (1986). Developing socio-dental indicators – the social impact of dental disease. *Community Dental Health* **3,** 3–17.
25. Shaw, W., Meek, S. and Jones, D. (1980). Nicknames, teasing, harassment and the salience of dental features amongst schoolchildren. *Brit. Journal Orthodontics,* **7,** 75–80.
26. Peter, J. and Chinsky, R. (1974). Sociological aspects of cleft palate adults I: marriage. *Cleft Palate Journal,* **11,** 259–309.
27. Smith, J. and Sheiham, A. (1979). How dental conditions handicap the elderly. *Community Dent. Oral Epidem.,* **7,** 305–310.
28. Baxter, J.C. (1981). Nutrition and the geriatric edentulous patient. *Spec. Care Dent.,* **1,** 259–261.
29. WHO (1977). Alma Ata Declaration. WHO, Geneva.
30. Tannahill, A. (1985). What is health promotion? *Health Education Journal,* **44,** 167–168. In: Downie, R.S., Fyfe, C. and Tannahill, A. (1990). *Health Promotion Models and Values.* Oxford Medical Publications.
31. Downie, R.S., Fyfe, C. and Tannahill, A. (1990). *Health Promotion Models and Values.* Oxford Medical Publications.
32. Milio N (1976) A framework for prevention: changing health damaging to health generating life patterns. *Am. J. Public Health,* **66,** 435–49.
33. Downie, R.S., Fyfe, C. and Tannahill, A. (1990). *Health Promotion Models and Values.* Oxford Medical Publications, p. 59.

18 Practical Oral Health Promotion

18.1 Introduction
18.2 Oral health promotion throughout life
18.3 The dependent child
18.4 The school student
18.5 Adulthood
18.6 Older age
18.7 Summary
18.8 References

18.1 Introduction

This chapter looks at practical ways in which oral health promotion can be undertaken in an integrated fashion, as part of the health promotion aspects of interventions.

18.2 Oral health promotion throughout life

An individual goes through a life career in certain roles, first as a dependent child, then a school student, next as an adult with differing roles, often including that of parent or carer, before passing into older age with a varying degree of dependence. As an individual passes through these stages, he or she is amenable at the time of transition to change, as part of taking on the new role. These changes present opportunities for health education that will be quickly accepted and acted on.

18.3 The dependent child

Health education activities
At this stage, health education involves giving information and skills to parents and carers on a healthy diet, oral hygiene methods, fluoride use, and early use of the dental services. As the dependent child has little opportunity to influence diet and to make informed choices, there is little educational value to be gained from targeting them without also including parents or carers.

A core oral health education message is that there is no role in a healthy diet for sugar (by which we mean non-milk extrinsic sugar). This message has to be conveyed as part of the promotion of a healthy diet. The method will vary in detail, but it should include alerting parents and carers to examine food labels for sugar content and to restrict sugar consumption to meal times only. The setting aside of specific times for eating confectionery is a practical strategy that many parents have found useful to counter the child's demands, and the pressures of advertising, grandparents and others who may encourage sugar consumption. Artificial and alternative sweeteners can be substituted for non-milk extrinsic sugars (Appendix 1).

Oral hygiene should be firmly tied into normal grooming and hygiene. The special techniques needed for an adult to carry out toothbrushing on a young child should be clearly taught and not assumed to be lay knowledge (Chapter 3). At this stage of life, it should be stressed that dental caries is neither normal nor inevitable. Similarly, it is important to stress that caries is caused by sugar in the diet and is not due to a lack of calcium, vitamin deficiency or an inherited condition, except in extremely rare cases.

Preventive activities
Health professionals involved in screening and health surveillance, should include the oral cavity, and seek early intervention by a dental professional, particularly for children at risk. Unfortunately, it is often still normal to wait until the tooth aches before seeking treatment, when dental pathology is advanced and restorative treatment is more difficult.

For carers, the application of fluoride in toothpaste or daily applied gels is an effective preventive activity as part of oral hygiene procedures.

Health protection
With the individual, positive health protection may involve encouraging values and attitudes that good oral health is attainable for virtually all children. This approach should avoid any 'victim blaming' where there has already been some oral disease. When advocating positive health, it is important to avoid becoming 'Utopian' and alienating the client.

18.4 The school student

This era of life is characterised by the learning that takes place in formal schooling and the growing influence of the peer group. Both these aspects present opportunities for health promotion.

Health education activities
Much of the school student's day is spent in a learning environment. The learning is often very structured and most school curricula include some

aspect of health education. Dental health education has always held a reasonably high profile in school-based health education, and traditionally health professionals have been involved. Health education has not only included dental health education, but also hygiene and sex education. Many countries are now adopting a new approach to health education in the curriculum.

Health education is being integrated across a range of subjects, reflecting the understanding that it concerns not only scientific facts, i.e. that sugar causes dental caries, but also wider issues such as the reasons that people consume sugar, despite knowing the health risk, and the existence of pressures in society to buy and consume sugar products. This broader understanding of health education has taken place alongside a recognition that most health education should be teacher-led and not by visiting specialists. The prolonged contact teachers have with their students allows them to reinforce and explore issues in a depth that the visiting specialist delivering a single lesson cannot hope to attain.

Many health professionals have had to consider the question, 'What is the role of the health professional in school-based health education?'. There is undoubtedly a role in supporting and advising the teacher. We have already touched on the concept that primary health professionals tend to be experts in their own fields and well-informed individuals in other health areas. The school teacher is in the same position. Most of us require extra guidance and support in this role.

It is therefore educationally sounder to leave the techniques and methods of education to the trained professional. The primary health care professional should concentrate on providing support and acting as a resource and advisor for the teacher. Many schools have now adopted policies regarding the role of the outside expert in the classroom, and most modern education is based on project based-learning which encourages the student to be active in seeking out the information.

The primary health care professional is likely to be most involved in helping the teacher during the time when school-term activities are planned. The teacher requires concise factual information and support, with resources and aids to learning. This involvement in cross-curricular teaching presents new challenges for the health professional. It is vital that we are adaptable to these new methods of teaching.

Preventive activities
In the UK, the school is a suitable venue for health surveillance, screening and epidemiological screening, including for dental and oral disease. Although this is currently delivered by dental professionals, the support of other primary health care professionals will greatly facilitate the procedure.

Carers of school students with special needs will be more directly involved in assisting with oral care on a daily basis. This may involve toothbrushing after meals and helping with the provision of oral care by the dental team.

Health protection

The school is not just for formal learning of specific subjects. There is also a lot of learning of morals, beliefs and attitudes, as part of the 'hidden curriculum'. It is important for effective learning that conflicting messages are not being presented by the wider school environment. The obvious example is the school snack-shop selling confectionery in contradiction to nutritional education, to supplement school funds. Most education authorities have now adopted a healthy eating policy for school meals, but the snack-shops are often a glaring loophole. The school environment should be health-promoting in all its aspects.

The primary health care professional can help by becoming involved in forming health policies and influencing the various decision-makers in the school. This includes not only the staff, but also school governors and parent associations.

18.5 Adulthood

This involves the work environment and parenthood, both areas requiring many life skills. The workplace is increasingly used as a venue for health promotion and issues such as safety, smoking, healthy eating and exercise.

Health education provided in the family setting is crucial for the health beliefs and behaviour of the child. Even though concepts of what constitutes a 'family' vary between different cultures and societies, we have taken the term to describe the environment in which a child grows and develops and is primary socialised.

The workplace

As an 'environment' rather than an age group is being discussed, it is more appropriate to consider the three areas of health promotion together. There have been advances in making the workplace more health-protective. This has involved health education at work, as well as direct preventive activities, such as health screening for coronary heart disease risk factors. It is important to reinforce the nutritional-based health promotion with sound oral practices. As the main oral risk for adults is periodontal disease, a health-promoting workplace should also provide facilities for workers to brush their teeth. It should also provide a suitable site for delivering health services, and the use of mobile facilities to provide dental care is gaining acceptance.

In all these aspects, the role of the primary health care professional is to initiate and facilitate these activities, and to influence those making decisions, whether management or staff associations.

The family

There is continuing discussion into where and how health promotion takes place in society, but it is widely accepted that most health education

Practical Oral Health Promotion

is given at home by women in their family role.[1] Parents receive knowledge and support from two main sources; these are different health professionals centred on the primary health care professional, and family and friends, collectively known as the 'lay system'. As described earlier, a person passes through several stages before making contact with professional dental services. These stages can be made easier by other health workers and carers acting as intermediaries and helping to break down barriers.

Most health care systems identify ante-natal, post-natal and early years in specific programmes. It is rarer for the dental team to be so intimately acquainted with the family at this stage.

Oral health education in the family

Much of what is relevant has already been covered in Chapter 3 on child dental health. The health professional can intervene to update and correct erroneous information, for example, adding sugar to bottle feeds to increase weight, dipping pacifiers in sugar or honey. Other misconceptions include the belief that white chocolate is a suitable safe confectionery for children, or that honey as a natural product is a safe alternative to sugar. It is the natural wish of all parents to provide the healthiest diet for their children and there are still misleading claims made by manufacturers. The recent growth in 'health drinks' with no added colorants, but with high sugar levels, is an oral health risk.

It is important to ensure that other environments also encourage good oral health. Unfortunately, this still includes other sectors of the health care system. Sweets continue to be given as a reward for good behaviour in many health facilities. A classic example is the polio vaccine delivered on a sugar lump!

18.6 Older age

The biological effects of ageing on oral tissues and the effects on oral health have already been explored in Chapter 4, but there are marked differences between the biological effects of ageing and those of 'social ageing'. This refers to the way in which factors in society influence the individual as to what is expected of them as an older person.

It is already known that demographic changes underway in industrialised northern countries will lead to relatively stable populations with an increasing average age. This is due to many social factors, such as better nutrition, housing and medical advances, resulting in increased life-expectancy, lower death rates, and the effects of the post-war 'baby boom'. However, the stereotypical picture still persists of older people as frail, dependent and edentulous. The oral health behaviour of much of the older population is characterised by low expectations of their oral health and low use of the dental services. Many of the aims of oral health promotion for this group are concerned with raising the expectations of individuals themselves, as well as those of the health professionals.

Health education activities

As with all groups, there are principles which the health educator should consider before tailoring programmes and activities to an individual's needs. With regard to older people, several broad principles have been identified[2]:

- Learning and recall are slower in older age and greater reinforcement of the messages, using spoken and written material, is important.
- Active learning in which individuals participate at their own pace is most likely to be successful.
- Written material should use larger print to facilitate reading.
- Older people get fatigued more easily and health education activities should be kept relatively short.

Older people have considerable life experience and have seen many changes in approaches to health. Initially, they may appear unwilling to change, and are more likely to rely on their own proven practice, until they see the personal value in change. Steel[3] has reviewed the relatively few oral health education programmes for older people. She noted that the most successful were those which employed behaviour modification techniques and did not concentrate purely on raising levels of knowledge. Several of the reviewed studies reported some success with peer group educators.

There are several pitfalls of which the oral health educator should be aware concerning older people. These involve the concept of 'ageism'[4] – negative attitudes to older people. These are common among health workers[5] and affect communication with older people. One result is a tendency to treat older people as children, particularly in communication. Dolinsky[6] describes this process as 'infantilisation' and says it will create barriers. It is worth stressing that even an older person suffering some degree of cognitive impairment or confusion may appear child-like in behaviour, but is still an adult with special needs.

The first step for the oral health educator is to gauge the impact of any oral disease, disability or ill-health on normal functioning, including social functioning. As described earlier, an easily usable measuring tool for oral health is not yet available, but sensitive, non-threatening questioning about physical, psychological and social functioning should reveal areas requiring action.

The core content of health education will vary depending on the oral status of that individual. For practical purposes, clients can be divided into dentate, partially dentate and edentulous. The last two groups may or may not be using a full or partial denture. The core knowledge the oral health educator requires will be found in Chapters 2 and 4. Modifications

Practical Oral Health Promotion

in oral hygiene and denture-cleaning techniques will need to be made depending on the presence of any functional disability, and it is useful to have suitable criteria for the individual to monitor their progress. Older people with a degree of dependence on a carer should also be included in the health education activity and common objectives agreed on.

An assessment of the oral health status of the carers or relatives will give insights into their oral care practices. Carers without formal training will employ their own practices and routines, including those for oral care. One study of oral care by non-professionally trained carers found that it was those carers with dentures who trained other carers and set the routines for oral care[7]. Even for highly dependent clients, self-care to whatever degree should be encouraged.

For the growing number of dentate older people, extra consideration needs to be given to their dietary practices. Taste and smell perception decrease with age and this may encourage an increase in sugar consumption. This and reduced saliva flow can place them at risk from root caries (see Chapter 4).

Preventive activities
A preventive role for the primary health care professional is to encourage regular screening for oral pathology. In common with the principles of involving the client in health-promoting practices, individuals should be encouraged to be aware of any early pathology, such as persistent ulcers or swellings. A parallel example is self-examination of the breasts for early breast pathology.

In the oral cavity, any ulcer that fails to heal after three weeks should be investigated. White or red patches on the oral mucosa may also be pre-malignant. It is the aim of the dental profession that all denture wearers should have an annual oral screening. However, it is not unusual for people to have worn dentures a decade or more and gradually adapted themselves to deficiencies in function and appearance.

For the dentate older person, the application of fluoride gels to exposed roots will help prevent root caries. Regular cleaning by a dental hygienist will help control periodontal disease.

Health protection
It is not unusual for aware oral health educators to find themselves in the position of countering ageism, as an effective health protection approach. Any environment, ward, centre or institution involved with older people, whether self-caring, dependent or semi-dependent for their everyday needs, should be a health-promoting environment. It is institutionalised ageism that will require combating. An excellent example is the provision of softer, almost minced foods. This legitimises masticatory problems and reduces the enjoyment of eating.

A problematic area for many older people is physical access to dental services. This is not just the dental office situated on the first floor without lift access, but the more intangible one of whether the whole ambience and approach is one which older people find comfortable. The effects of ageing on sensory and auditory processes can make the dental environment more threatening.

The primary health professional, who is most acquainted with an individual's needs, can reduce the barriers by pre-planning with the dental services. For the relative minority of older people who have insurmountable physical access problems, oral care can often be provided in the home environment, and can be facilitated via the primary health care team.

Oral health promotion for this broad group presents many challenges, due to the need for all institutions in society, including health care institutions, to reassess their perceptions of the older person. Demographic and other changes mean that older people are living longer, are healthier and more independent, and are challenging their traditional stereotypes. These changes include their oral health status.

18.7 Summary

There are certain key stages during life at which oral health promotion can be maximised. These are the early years, school age, adulthood and older age. Effective oral health promotion for all these stages consists of a combination of health education, prevention and health protection. At all stages, the input of primary health care professionals is important, as they have a closer contact with the client than the dental team. See also Appendix 1 for details of resources for oral health promotion and information on sugar substitutes.

18.8 References

1. Graham, H. (1984). Women, Health and the Family. In: Rodmell, S. and Watt, A. (Eds.) 1986. *The Politics of Health Education*. London, Wheatsheaf Books.
2. Kiyak, A. (1984). Utilisation of dental services by the elderly. *Gerodontology*, **3**, 17–25.
3. Steel, L. (1989). *A Participative Approach to Oral Health*. London, Health Education Authority, p. 19.
4. Brock, A.M. (1985). Communicating with the elderly patient. *Spec. Care in Dent.*, **5**, 157–159.
5. Steel, L. (1989). *A Participative Approach to Oral Health*. London, Health Education Authority, p. 21.
6. Dolinsky, E.H. and Dolinsky, H.B. (1983). Infantilisation of elderly patients by health care providers. *Spec. Care in Dent.*, **4**, 150–153.
7. Boyle, S.J. (1992). Assessing Oral Care. *Nursing Times*, **88**(15), 44–48.

Appendix 1: Resource Addresses

Resources for oral health promotion
The most valuable resource for effective health promotion is the human resource! For those health professionals who have a direct role in promoting oral health sources of information and access to aids, learning will be useful.

Sources of local and regional information
For information on availability of dental services, information on local oral health needs:

- Family Health Service Authority.
- Director of Dental Public Health.
- The Local Community Dental Service may already be involved in oral health promotion programmes.
- District Health Promotion Unit.

For regional information in the UK on dental services and advice on oral health education material:

- Action and Information on Sugar, c/o 57 Turner St, London, E1 2AD.
- British Dental Association, 64 Wimpole St, London, W1M 8DQ.
- British Dental Health Foundation, 88 Gurnards Avenue, Fishermead, Milton Keynes, MK6 2BL.
- British Fluoridation Society, 64 Wimpole St, London, W1M 8DQ.
- General Dental Council, 37 Wimpole St, London, W1M 8DQ.
- Health Education Authority, Hamilton House, Mabledon Place, London, WC1H 9TX.
- Health Promotion Wales, Ffynnon Las, Tyglas Ave, Llanishen, Cardiff, CF4 5DZ; tel. 0222 752222.
- Health Education Board for Scotland, Health Education Centre, Woodburn House, Canaan Lane, Edinburgh, E10 4SG.
- London Food Commission, 88 Old St, London, EC1V 9AR.
- Northern Ireland Health Promotion Unit, The Beeches, 12 Hampton Manor Drive, Belfast, BT7 3EN.

Resource and programme information
Your Local Community Dental Service may be able to offer help with resources they have developed. Some manufacturers also offer resources but these should be evaluated carefully before use. The largest manufacturers include:

- ClinicAid Ltd, University Innovation Centre, Singleton Park, Swansea, West Glamorgan, SA2 8PP.
- Colgate Hoyt Professional Dental Service, Red Lion House, High St, High Wycombe, Buckinghamshire, HP11 2BX.
- Cooper Health Products, Gatehouse Rd, Aylesbury, Buckinghamshire, HP19 3ED.
- Gibbs Hygiene Service, Hesketh House, Portman Square, London, W1A 1DY.
- Hemming Visual Aid Ltd., 122 Bailiff St, Northampton, NN1 3EA.
- Imperial Chemical Industries Plc., Pharmaceutical Division, Alderley House, Alderley, Macclesfield, SK10 4TF.
- Johnson & Johnson, Dental Care Division, Brunel Way, Slough, Berkshire, SL1 1XR.
- Macleans, Dental Health and Education Services, Beecham House, Great West Rd, Brentford, Middlesex, TW8 9BD.
- Proctor and Gamble Ltd., Professional Services Division, PO Box 1EP, Newcastle upon Tyne, NE99 1EP.
- Stafford Miller, The Common, Hatfield, Herts, AL10 ONZ.
- Sterling Health, 1 Onflow St, Guildford, GU1 4YS.
- Unilever Scottish Central Film Library, Dowanhill, 74 Victoria Crescent, Glasgow, G12 9JN.

Alternatives to non-milk extrinsic sugars

Although there will be variations in the availability of artificial sweeteners under additive legislation between countries, the commonest include:

- **Saccharin**: This is 200 to 500 times sweeter than sucrose, but sometimes has an unpleasant aftertaste. It is heat-stable and used widely in food and beverage preparation.
- **Acesulfame K**: This is 200 times sweeter than sucrose. It is not metabolised and is stable in food preparations. It has less aftertaste than saccharin.
- **Aspartame**: This is 200 times sweeter than sucrose and has virtually no metabolic value. It loses its taste in cooking and is thus used primarily in beverages or uncooked food.
- **Cylamate**: This is 30 times sweeter than sucrose and is heat-stable. Often used in combination with saccharin. Currently not available in USA or UK.
- **Alternative sugars**: These modified sugars yield the same energy value as sucrose but are acceptable to people with diabetes and are not cariogenic. They include sorbitol, isomalt, mannitol, xylitol and hydrogenated glucoses, and are used in paediatric medicines and in some confectionery.

Appendix 2: Disabled Living Centres

These provide a valuable source of professional information and advice on independent living, and will be able to give specific advice on aids to personal care. All centres are fully accessible and open at regular advertised times during the week. Most use an appointment system to ensure that visitors get the best from the services available, but will do their best to accomodate casual visitors. For further information contact the Disabled Living Centres Council, telephone 071 266 2059.

Aberdeen
Hillylands Disabled Living Centre,
Croft Road,
Mastrick,
Aberdeen, AB2 6RB
Tel. 0224 685247

Aylesbury
Stoke Mandeville Independent
Living Exhibition,
Stoke Mandeville Hospital,
Mandeville Road,
Aylesbury,
Bucks, HP21 8AL.
Tel. 0296 84111 x3114

Belfast
Disabled Living Centre,
Regional Disablement Services,
Musgrave Park Hospital,
Stockman's Lane,
Belfast, BT9 7JB.
Tel. 0232 669501 x2708

Birmingham
Disabled Living Centre,
260 Broad Street,
Birmingham,
B1 2HF.
Tel. 021 643 0980

Bodelwyddan
North Wales Resource Centre for
Disabled People,
Ysbyty Glan Clwyd,
Bodelwyddan,
Clwyd, LL18 5UJ.
Tel. 0745 583910 x4706/4609

Braintree
Independent Living Advice
Centre,
Black Notley Hospital,
Braintree, Essex.
Tel. 0376 21068

Caerphilly
Resources (Aids and Equipment)
Centre,
Wales Council for the Disabled,
'Llys Ifor',
Crescent Road,
Caerphilly,
Mid-Glamorgan, CF8 1XL.
Tel. 0222 887325/6/7

Cardiff
Disabled Living Centre,
The Lodge,
Rookwood Hospital,
Fairwater Road,
Llandaff,
South Glamorgan, CF5 2YN.
Tel. 0222 566281 x3751

Holistic Oral Care

Carmarthen
Cwm Disability Centre for
Independent Living,
Coomb House,
Hangynog,
Carmarthen,
Dyfed, SA33 5HP.
Tel. 0267 83743

Colchester
Disabled Living Centre,
Occupational Therapy Dept
Colchester General Hospital,
Colchester.
Tel. 0206 853535 x2172/2173

Edinburgh
Lothian Disabled Living Centre,
Astley Ainslie Hospital,
Grange Loan,
Edinburgh, EH9 2HL.
Tel. 031 447 6271 x5635

Exeter
Independent Living Centre,
St. Loye's School of Occupational
Therapy,
Millbrook House,
Topsham Road,
Exeter, EX2 6ES.
Tel. 0392 59260

Huddersfield
Disabled Living Centre,
Kirklees Social Services,
Unit 6, Silvercourt Trading Estate,
Silver Street,
Huddersfield, West Yorks.
Tel. 0482 28631 x332

Hull
St. Hilda House,
National Demonstration Centre,
Kingston General Hospital,
Beverley Road,
Hull, HU3 1UR.
Tel. 0482 28631 x332

Inverness
Disabled Living Centre,
Raigmore Hospital,
Inverness, IV2 3UJ.
Tel. 0463 234151 x293

Leeds
The William Merritt Disabled
Living Centre,
St. Mary's Hospital,
Greenhill Road,
Leeds, LS12 3QE.
Tel. 0532 793140

Leicester
The Disabled Living Centre,
British Red Cross Medical Aid Dept
76 Clarendon Park Road,
Leicester, LE2 3AD.
Tel. 0533 700747

Liverpool
Merseyside Centre for
Independent Living,
Youens Way,
East Prescot Road,
Liverpool, L14 2EP.
Tel. 051 228 9221

London
The Disabled Living Foundation,
380/384 Harrow Road,
London, W9 2HU.
Tel. 071 289 6111

Macclesfield
Disabled Living Centre,
Macclesfield District General
Hospital,
Victoria Road,
Macclesfield,
Cheshire, SK10 3BL.
Tel. 0625 661740

Manchester
Regional Disabled Living Centre,
Disabled Living Services,
Redbank House,
4 St. Chad's Street,
Cheetham,
Manchester, M8 8QA.
Tel. 061 832 3678

Middlesbrough
Department of Rehabilitation,
Middlesbrough General Hospital,
Ayresome Green Lane,
Middlesbrough,
Cleveland, TS5 5AZ.
Tel. 0642 850222 x158

Newcastle upon Tyne
Newcastle upon Tyne Council For the Disabled,
The Dene Centre,
Castles Farm Road,
Newcastle upon Tyne, NE3 1PH.
Tel. 091 284 0480

Nottingham
Nottingham Resource Centre for the Disabled,
Lenton Business Centre,
Lenton Boulevard,
Nottingham, NG7 2BY.
Tel. 0602 420391

Paisley
Disability Centre for Independent Living,
Community Services Centre,
Queen Street,
Paisley, Strathclyde.
Tel. 041 887 0597

Portsmouth
The Frank Sorrell Centre,
Prince Albert Road,
Eastney, Portsmouth, PO4 9HR.
Tel. 0705 737174

Semington
Western Wiltshire Disabled Living Centre,
St. George's Hospital,
Semington,
Wiltshire, BA14 6JQ.
Tel. 0380 871007

Southampton
Southampton Aid and Equipment Centre,
Southampton General Hospital,
Tremona Road,
Southampton, SO9 4XY.
Tel. 0703 796631

Stockport
Disabled Living Centre,
St. Thomas' Hospital,
Shawheath,
Stockport, Cheshire, SK3 8BL.
Tel. 061 419 4476

Swansea
Disabled Living Assessment Centre,
St. John's Road,
Manselton,
Swansea, SA5 8PR.
Tel. 0792 580161

Swindon
The Swindon Centre for Disabled Living,
The Hawthorn Centre,
Cricklade Road,
Swindon, Wiltshire, SN2 1AF.
Tel. 0793 643966

Welwyn Garden City
Easier Living Exhibitions,
Herts Assoc for the Disabled,
The Woodside Centre,
The Commons,
Welwyn Garden City,
Hertfordshire, AL7 4DD.
Tel. 0707 324581

Holistic Oral Care

DAI (Disabled Advice and Information)
Mobile touring exhibition:
Wales Council for the Disabled,
'Llys Ifor',
Crescent Road,
Caerphilly,
Mid-Glamorgan, CF8 1XL.
Tel. 0222 887325/6/7

MAC (Mobile Advice Centre)
Mobile touring exhibition:
Disability Scotland,
Princes House,
5 Shandwick Place,
Edinburgh, EH2 4RG.
Tel. 031 229 8632

Further Reading

Andlaw, R.J. and Rock, W.P. (1982). *A Manual of Paedodontics*. Churchill Livingstone.
Besford, J. (1984). *Good Mouthkeeping*. Oxford University Press.
Blinkhorn, A.S., Fox, B. and Holloway, P. (1980). *Notes for Students of Dental Health Education*. 2nd Ed. Health Education Authority.
COMA (1989). *Dietary Sugars and Human Disease*. Report 37. COMA panel. Education Authority. HMSO.
Cook, R. and Cook, E. (1983). *Sugar Off*. Pan.
Coote, B. (1987). *The Hunger Crop*. Oxfam.
Davis, P. (1987). *Introduction to the Sociology of Dentistry*. Otago Press.
Downie, R.S., Fyfe, C. and Tannahill, A. (1990). *Health Promotion Models and Values*. Oxford University Press.
Elderton, R.J. (1987). *Positive Dental Prevention*. Heinemann Press.
Elderton, R.J. (1988). *The Dentition in Health and Disease*. Wright.
Ewles L. and Simnett I. (1992). *Promoting Health*. 2nd Ed. Scutari.
Griffiths, J.E. (1991). The Dental Needs of the Elderly and the Delivery of Care. In: *Principles and Practice of Geriatric Medicine* Pathy, M.S.J. (ed.) 2nd Ed. Wiley.
Hunter, B. (1987). *Dental Care for Handicapped Patients*. Wright.
Jacob, M.J. and Plamping, D. (1989). *The Practice of Primary Dental Care*. Wright.
Locker, D. (1989). *Behavioural Science & Dentistry*. Routledge.
Royal College of Physicians. (1976). *Fluoride Teeth and Health*. A Report of the Royal College of Physicians. Pitman Medical.
Scully, C. (1985). *Hospital Dental Surgeon's Guide*. Latimer.
Scully, C. and Cawson, R.A. (1987). *Medical Problems in Dentistry*. 2nd Ed. Wright.
Slack, G.L. and Burt, B.A. (1985). *Dental Public Health*. 2nd Ed. Wright.
Yudkin, J. (1986). *Pure, White and Deadly*. Penguin.

Glossary

Abrasion: Wear of enamel usually by incorrect toothbrushing.

Angular cheilitis: Chronic infection of the corners of the mouth.

Bottle caries: Dental caries of the primary dentition, usually the front teeth. Caused by drinking sugar containing drinks from a bottle, often at night.

Bridgework: A fixed appliance to replace a missing tooth or teeth

Bruxism: Grinding of teeth, often nocturnal.

Calculus: Calcified deposit found on teeth, usually near to ducts of salivary glands and acts as a plaque trap.

Cariogenic: A sugar that has the potential to provoke dental caries.

Cementum: The outer layer of the root of a tooth to which are attached the periodontal membranes.

Chronic inflammatory periodontal disease: Often known as 'gum disease'. The disease process that results in destruction of the periodontal membrane, loss of bony support and subsequent mobility and loss of teeth.

Cortical bone: The outer, denser layer of jaw bone.

Crowns: Either the visible part of the tooth in the mouth or refers to the artificial porcelain or metal replacement cemented to the tooth.

Demineralisation: The loss of mineral from the enamel surface when the environment becomes acidic following ingestion of sugar.

Dental caries: The loss of mineral, production of a cavity and destruction of the tooth caused by the action of sugar with dental plaque.

Dental plaque: A colony of bacteria in a cellular substrate which forms on teeth.

Dentate: Possessing natural teeth.

Dentine: The mineralised substance that forms the bulk of the tooth underneath the harder enamel outer coat.

Denture sore mouth: A euphemism as it not usually sore. Chronic candidosis seen on the mucosa under a denture.

Disclosing tablets: Vegetable dye, usually red used to stain dental plaque to aid effective toothbrushing.

DMFT: Decayed, Missing and Filled Teeth; an index used in dental surveys.

Edentulous: The state of not possessing natural teeth.

Glossary

Enamel: The hard outer layer of the tooth.

Erosion: The loss of enamel by prolonged contact with acidic solutions, often fruit juices.

Fixed appliances: Usually orthodontic appliances bonded to the teeth. Can also refer to splints used following jaw surgery.

Fluoride: A naturally occuring mineral which prevents dental caries by increasing resistance of the enamel to demineralisation.

Fluorosis: Mottling, white or brown patches seen on enamel due to high ingestion of fluoride during the formation of the enamel.

Gingival hyperplasia: overgrowth of gum tissue. Can be the result of chronic irritation or generalised as a side effect of some drugs, e.g. Epanutin.

Gingiva: The margin of the gum in contact with the crown of the tooth.

Gingivitis: Inflammatory condition of the gum caused by dental plaque.

Glossitis: Inflammation of the tongue. Can be caused by certain drugs or vitamin deficiency.

Hypercementosis: Proliferation of the cementum of the root, which complicates dental extractions.

Implantology: A new technique to replace extracted teeth with titanium implants to support a crown or denture.

Incisors: Front teeth used for cutting.

Intermaxillary fixation: An oral surgery technique for imobilising jaw fractures by splinting to the opposite jaw.

Interproximal: The zone between teeth, difficult to clean effectively and a site where caries and gum disease can start.

Leukoplakia: a white patch in the oral cavity which may be pre-malignant.

Malocclusions: An abnormal relationship between upper and lower jaws.

Molars: Back teeth used for grinding and chewing.

Mottling: White or brown patches on enamel, *see* **fluorosis.**

Mucositis: A serious inflammation of the mucosa seen in patients undergoing chemotherapy and radiotherapy.

Occlusal: The flat, chewing surface of molar teeth.

Oral mucosa: Mucous membranes lining the mouth.

Oral hypersensitivity: A reaction of the oral mucosa which may be drug related.

Orthodontics: Treatment of malocclusions with fixed and removable appliances.

Holistic Oral Care

Periodontal fibres: Supporting fibres connecting the tooth to the bone.

Periodontal disease: Also known as 'gum disease'. Chronic inflammatory disease affecting periodontal fibres and bony support caused by dental plaque.

Primary dentition: First set of teeth (20) which erupt in the first few months and are replaced.

Pulp tissue: The central, living core of the tooth composed of blood vessels and nervous tissue.

Secondary dentition: Second set of teeth (32) which start to erupt at 6 years of age.

Sinusitis: Inflammation of the membranes lining the maxillary sinuses, can be confused with toothache.

Stomatitis: Inflammation of the mucosa.

Tartar: A commonly used name for **calculus**.

Tempero-mandibular joint (TMJ): The joint between the lower jaw and the skull.

Trigeminal neuralgia: A condition which produces severe facial pain.

Xerostomia: A dry mouth, the result of reduced salivary flow.

Index

Page numbers in bold type indicate an illustration or table occurs on this page.

A

access
   to information 63, 68, 128, 132
   to services 61, 68, 128, 132, 141, 152
acid
   high food content **32**
   in caries 11–12, 13, 24, 27, 30, 31
   reduction 32
   regurgitation 32, 142–3, 177, **191**
acquired bleeding disorders 108, **189**
acute renal failure 89
adolescents
   psychiatric disease 179–80
age
   barriers to dental care 61–6
   community dental services 78
   dementia 172–3
   dental health 60–1
   disability 57–8
   oral care 64–8
   oral effects 58–60
   oral health promotion 245–8
   oral status 60
   psychosis 176–7
   routine check-ups 64
   see also social ageing
AIDS 173, 199–201
akinesia 140
alcoholic heart muscle disease 184
allogeneic transplants 210
aluminium 173
Alzheimer's disease 172–4
anaemia 133, 157, 178, **186**–8, 191, 206, 210
anaesthesia *see* general anaesthesia
angina 184
angular cheilitis 191, 196
anorexia nervosa 177–8
anti-coagulant therapy 182–93
anti-hypertensives
   oral side-effects 110, **183**
anti-plaque effect 66, 119, 120
antibacterial
   effects of saliva 107
   thymol activity 120
antibiotic cover 182–93
anticholinesterase 137

anticonvulsant drugs 110, 143, 147–8, 158, 160
antipsychotic medication
   side-effects 110, **164**
anxiety
   barriers to dental care 62, 167
aplastic anaemia 187
appliances
   oral care 36–8, 39, 66–7, 96, 123–4
appointments
   child dental health 52
arthritis 133–4, **134**
aspirating toothbrushes **115**
assessment
   chemotherapy 209
   child dental health 44–5
   guides 1–2, **90**
   high-risk 47
   key indicators 88
asthma **190**
at-risk
   child dental health 42–3
   groups 2, 127–30, 151–61, 208
   individuals 45–**7**
atherosclerotic dementia 173
atropic candidiasis 196
atropine 137
attendance patterns 63
autism
   risk factors 159
autologous transplants 210

B

bacteraemia 156, 186, 206
bacterial
   endocarditis 142
   plaque reduction 119
barriers
   dental care 61–4, 152–3
   oral health 132, 165
battery-operated toothbrushes 114
Behçet's syndrome 191
Bell's palsy 139
benzhexol 140
benzydamine hydrochloride 121
bleeding disorders 188–9
blood disorders *see* dyscrasias

Index

BMT transplantation **215**
bone 7, 9, 133, 134, 135
   deformity 136
   effects of aging 59
   marrow transplants 118, 120, 188, 210–11, **211**
borate toxicity 120
bridges
   care of appliances 36–8
British Dental Association 34, 118
brittle bone disease *see* osteogenesis imperfecta
bromocriptine 140
bruxism 142, 169
bulimia 177–8
burning mouth syndrome 169, 188
butyrophenones 139

C

calcium deficiency 135
calculus 8, 37
   removal 9, 39, 81
candidiasis 194–6, **195**, 200
carbamazepine 138, 148
carcinoma *see* oral carcinoma
cardiac abnormalities 134, 184
cardiomyopathies 184
cardiovascular diseases 182–6
carers 85–6
caries *see* dental caries
cerebral palsy 119, 129, 141–**3**
   risk factors 158
cerebrovascular accident 138–9
cetylpyridinium chloride 119
charges 62, 75–6
chemical burns 108
chemical plaque control 66, 119, 160
chemotherapy 89, 208–9, **215**
child dental health 42–55
   assessment 44–5
   dentitions 43–4
   evaluation 53
   holistic approach to prevention 45–7
   implementation of preventive regimes 48
   oral preventive strategy process 44
   primary prevention 43
   psychiatric disease 179–80
   special needs 42–3
   toothbrushes 113
chlorhexidine gluconate 111, 119, 160, 202, 206, 214, 215

gel 96, 119, 214
   mouthwash 96, 119, 202, 206, 214, 221
   spray 119, 143
chronic
   hyperplastic candidiasis 196
   inflammatory periodontal disease 7–9
chronically sick children 108
cleaners
   denture care 38, **39**
CLAPA 141
cleft lip and palate 140–1
client's views
   assessment 91–4, **94**
coeliac disease 191
coloured filaments 113
COMA report **25**, **26**
Committee on the Safety of Medicines 120
Community Dental Services 77–8
   domiciliary dental care 80, 174
congenital
   bleeding disorders 188–9
   heart disease 156, 184
contact reactions 108
continuing care 73–4
Court Report 154
Creutzfeldt–Jakob syndrome 173
Crohn's disease 191
cross infection control
   HIV infection 202–3
cultural barriers 63–4
cystic fibrosis 190
cytomegaloviral infection 184
cytotoxics **207**, **212**

D

decay
   elderly status 60–1
   factors 11–12
   process **10**
delayed eruption 141, 184
delirium 171
dementia **172**
dental
   care
     age barriers 61–4
     learning disability barriers 152–3
   caries 9–13
     cause 11
     children **17**
     distribution 15–17
     factors affecting dental decay 11–12

Index

hygienists 81, 147
learning disabilities 153–4
methods of plaque control 13
prevention 13, 27–9, 30
rate **15**
role of toothbrushing 12
signs and symptoms of dental caries 11
trends **16**
disease
  child dental health 46–7
floss **30**, 115–**16**
health
  learning disabilities 153–4
  mental illness 162–81
  older people 60–1
prevention **27–9**
teaching hospitals 78–9
therapists 80–1
dentitions
  primary and secondary 43–4
dentures
  care 37, 66–7, 96, 123, 124
  cleaning aids **39**, 123, **124**
  related conditions 60–1
  use and abuse 38–40
  see also naming dentures
dependency 105, 129
dependent individual
  aspirating toothbrushes 115
  child health education 241–2
  oral
    assessment 95–6, **96**
    care 220–**221**
depressive neuroses 168
desensitisation 118
diabetes 192–3
  insipidus 192
  mellitus 192–3
dietary care
  acid control 32
  changes
    child dental health 48
  COMA report **25**
  sugar reduction 24–7
disabilities
  age **57**–60
  learning 151–61
  oral handicap 18–19, 234–5
  physical and mental 46, 162–81
disabled groups
  adaptations 122
  electric toothbrushes 114
  mouthrinses 119

Disabled Living
  Centres 124, 251–4
  Foundation 122
disclosing materials 113
disease *see* oral disease
distribution of oral disease 15–18
  dental caries 15–17
  periodontal disease 17
  tooth loss 17–18
District Health Authorities 132
domiciliary dental care 80, 174
dopamine 139
double-headed toothbrush 113–**14**
Down's syndrome 140
  learning skills 157–**8**
  oral abnormalities 155–**6**
  physiological factors 156–**7**
  risk factors 154–5, 184
drooling 140
drugs
  induced blood disorders 108
  pregnancy 108
  risk factors 159–60
  side-effects 108–9, 133, **134**, 140
dry mouth *see* xerostomia
dyscrasias 108, 186–8
dysphagia 138
  causes 218–220
dysphagic patients
  aspirating toothbrushes 115, 221
  causes **218**–220
  oral care **220**–221

E

eating disorders **177**
  symptoms 178
economic barriers to dental care 62
edentulous status 60
education
  nursing team 100–1
  oral health promotion **236**–9, 241–8
electric toothbrushes 114
emotional handicap 77
environmental factors 112
epidemiological screening 243
epiglottis oedema 120
epilepsy 141, 147–**8, 172**
  risk factors 158
Epstein–Barr virus 196–8
equipment **95**
evaluation
  child dental health 53
extractions

261

Index

elderly status 60–1
primary teeth 81
extrinsic sugars **26**, 107

F

facial
  dyskinesia 140, 170, 176
  paralysis 138
  prostheses 38
Fanconi's anaemia 187–8
Family Health Services Authority 76–7, 132
family oral health promotion 244–5
fear
  barriers to dental care 62
FHSA 76–7
filaments 113
fillings 81
fixation
  care of appliances 36–7
  oral dependency 105
flossing tapes **30**, 115–**16**
fluoride products 118
  application 81, 178, 237
  child dental care 50–2
  dosage schedule **31**
  oral care 31–2
  rinse 118
flycatcher tongue 140
foam sticks 113, 117
foetal development 108
folic acid deficiency 187
food allergies 113

G

gastrointestinal disease 191
gauze strips 117
general
  anaesthesia 182–93
  dental practitioners 73–7
    domiciliary dental care 80
genetic influences on aging 58
geographical location
  child dental health 46
  community dental services 77
gingival bleeding 188
glandosane 121
glycerine swabs 121
graft versus host disease **211**
gram-positive bacteria 119
Gilles de la Tourette's syndrome 159
gingival irritation 118

Guillain–Barré syndrome 138
gum
  care 33–5
  disease 60–1
GVHD 210

H

habits 58
haemolytic anaemias 188
haemophilia 188
haemorrhage risk 188
hairy leukoplakia 200
handicap *see* disability
HBV infection **198**
head injuries **146**–7
Health for All 2000 declaration 236
health
  behaviour 231–2
  child dental 42–55
  education 237–9, 241–8
  educator training 82
  illness behaviour 230–1
  oral 3, 6–22, 13, 19–20, 60–1, 64–8, 229–30
  perceptions 229–30
  potential 232–3
  promotion 235–9, **236**, 241–8
  status 233–4
hearing impairment 149
hemiplegia 105, 138
hepatitis virus 198
herpes simplex I and II 196–7
hexetidine 118, 119
high-risk assessment
  child dental health 47
history 71–3
HIV
  gingivitis 200
  infection 173, 195, 199–**200**
  periodontitis 200
  -related conditions 201
holistic approach
  attitudes 129
  child dental health 45–7
hormone deficiencies 135
hospital
  dental services 78
  toothbrushes 113
Huntington's chorea 173
hydrocephalus 143–4
hydrogen peroxide 120
hygiene
  aids 117, 221–2

care of appliances 38
child dental care 49–52
malignant disease 213, **214**
medically compromised patients 182–93
hygienist training 81
hypertension 183
Hypromellose 121
hysterical neuroses 167–8

I

ICU patients 89, **91**
idiopathic cardiomyopathies 184
illness behaviour 230–1
immunosuppressive therapy **185**, 211, **212**
impaired reflexes 142
swallow *see* dysphagia
implementation
preventive regimes for children 48
in-patients dental services 79
Independent Living Centres 112
infantilisation 246
infective endocarditis 156, 189–93, **186**
information
dental services 63
interdental brushes 116, **117**
intrinsic sugars **26**
iron deficiency 187
irrigation devices 116–17
ischaemic heart disease 184
isotonic saline 121

J

jaw
abnormal development 155
dislocation 142
pain 184
juvenile arthritis 134

K

Kaposi's sarcoma 201
key stressors 88
kidney disease 192
Korsakoff's syndrome 179

L

laryngeal oedema 120
learning disabilities
community dental care 77
oral and dental problems 151–61, 179

lemon swabs 121
Lesch–Nyhan syndrome 159
leukaemia 188, 206–7
leukoplakia 173
levodopa 140
lifestyle effects of aging 58
lithium 171
liver disease 192
Luborant 121
lymphoblastic leukaemia **206**

M

mains-operated toothbrushes 114
malaria 188
malignant disease
diagnosis 207
oral care 35, 212–14
oral complications of treatment 207–12
treatment 205–16
malocclusions 136, 141
malpositioned teeth 115, 184
manic psychosis 170–1
manual toothbrushes 113–14
maxillofacial surgery 207–8
medical conditions
child dental health 46
community dental services 77
medications
anti-psychotic side-effects 165
application 81
oral side effects **110–11**, 159–60, 165–66
medicines
sugar content 107–8, 141, 159–60, 184
mental
disabilities
child dental health 46
community dental service 77
handicap 77, 151–61, 179
illness 162–181
behavioural factors **165**
micro-organisms 107
mobility
barriers to dental care 61, 128
molar tootth **8**
motor neurone disease 137
mouth appliances 124–5
mouthcare 35, 66
mouthwashes 118–21
MRSA 195
mucosal irritation 120
mucositis 208

263

Index

mucosolvents 120
multidisciplinary oral care 101–2, 139
multiple sclerosis 137–8
muscular dystrophy 136–7
    Becker type 136
    Duchenne type 136
myasthenia gravis 137
myeloblastic leukaemia 206
myelosuppression 211
myotonic disorders 136–7

N

naming dentures
    care of appliances 39–40, 68
narcotics addiction 179
neuroses 166–9
neurosyphilis 173
neutral pH fluoride preparations 118
NHS dental care 73–7
non-Hodgkin's lymphoma 201
NSAIDs 133
nurse manager
    oral care promotion 99–106
nurses 85–6
nursing guides **90**
nutritional effects on aging 58

O

observed behaviour 89–91
obsessional neuroses 168
obturators
    care of appliances 38
occasional patients 74
occlusal and proximal surfaces **12**
OPCS survey **57**
oral
    assessment 1–2, **44**–5
        guide for nursing assistants **90**, **92–3**
        outcomes 94
        systems 89
    carcinoma 13–15, 187
        diagnosis 207–8
        risk factors 14–15
    care 23–41, 129
        appliance care 36–8
        dementia 174
        dental caries prevention 13, 27–9, 30
        denture use and abuse 38–40
        dependent patients 220–**1**
        dietary control 24–7, 32
        dysphagic patients 220–1
        factors **41**

fluoride products **31**–2
gum care 33–5
malignant disease 35, 212–15, **214, 215**
mental illness 162–81
mouth care 35
older people 56–70, **65**
nurse manager's role 99–106
plaque control 13, 27–9, 30
terminal illness 222–3
tooth care 24
see also practical oral care
disability 234–5
disease 7
    COMA report **25**
    distribution 15–18
    effects on aging 58
    medically compromised patients 182–93
see also malignant disease
health and disease 6–22
    global oral health trends **18**
health promotion
    approaches and practices 3, 225–40
    diet sheets **27–9**
    eating disorder symptoms **178**
    HIV infection 201–3
    learning disabilities 151–61
    mental illness 163–5
    practical 241–8
    prevention 19–20, **44**–5, **160**
    strategy development 100
hygiene measures
    aids 117
    child dental health 49–50, 50–2
irrigation devices 116–17
radiotherapy complications **209**
self-care 112–26
self-mutilation 159
side-effects 133, **134**, 137, **140, 206**–7
tissues
    effects of aging 59
    ulceration 191
organic cerebral disorders 171
orodental needs 88
orofacial complaints 168
orphenadrine 140
orthodontic appliances 36, 115
osteitis deformans 136
osteoarthritis 133
osteogenesis imperfecta 134–5
osteomalacia 135
osteoporosis 135
Ottawa Charter 229
oxygenating agents 120

P

pacemakers 184
Paget's disease *see* osteitis deformans
Parkinson's disease 139–40
  side-effects **140**, 176
parotid salivery glands 188
Pat Saunders drinking straw 124
periodontal disease 7–9
  distribution 17
  learning disabilities 153–4
personality disorders 167
pharmacotherapy 107
PHCA 228
phenol 120
phenothiazines 139
phenytoin 138, 147
phobias 167
psychiatric drugs 139, 163–5
psychosomatic disorders 177
physical disabilities 131–50
  child dental health 46
  community dental services 77
  prevalence 132
Pica syndrome 159
Pick's disease 173
pipe cleaners 117
plaque control 13, 27–9, 30
  chemical 66, 118–19, 142, 206
  detection 113
  learning disabilities 151–61
  removal 117–18
povidone iodine 120
practical oral care 1, 5–84
practice information 74–5
pregnancy 108
prevention
  child dental health 43, 44–53
  dental caries 13, 27–9, 30
  oral disease 19–20
    primary 19
    secondary 20
    tertiary 20
preventive health
  education 237–9, 241–8
  learning disabilities **160**–1
  medically compromised patients 182–93
  services 237
  primary
  health care 228–9
  herpetic gingivostomitis 196–7
private dental treatment 75
Project 2000 229
prothrombin times (INR) 183

pseudomembranous candidiasis 195
psychiatric disease
  child dental health 179–80
  medication risk factors 163–4
psychoses 169–77
  in older people 176–7

R

radiation treatment 118, 208
radiotherapy 209–10, **215**
rechargeable toothbrushes 114
removable appliances
  care 37–8
renal insufficiency 120
reported behaviour 89–91
research 86
resource addresses 249–50
respiratory disorders 189–90
rheumatic heart disease 184
rheumatoid arthritis 133
rickets 135
Riley–Day syndrome 159
routine check-ups 64
rubella 184

S

saliva
  effects of aging 59
  oral health 13
  Orthana 121
  substitutes 121
scaling 81
schizophrenia 175–6
school students
  oral health promotion 242–4
screening 243
secondary herpes simplex infection 196–7
self-caring individuals
  aids 112–26
  oral assessment **95**
self-mutilation *see* oral self-mutilation
self-pasting toothbrushes 123
sensory impairment 148–9
services 73–7
  future developments 82–3
sickle-cell disease 188
sickness impact profile categories **233**
side-effects of drugs 108–9
single-tufted toothbrushes **114**–15
Sjögren's syndrome 133
social ageing 245–8
socially disadvantaged people

Index

community dental services 77
sodium
    bicarbonate 120
    chloride 121
    fluoride solution 118
    perborate 120
special needs see at-risk groups
spina bifida 143–4
spinal injuries and trauma 144–**5**
squamous cell carcinoma 207
St. Vitus dance 184
stannous fluoride solution 118
steroid therapy 133, 137, 207, 211–12
Still's disease 134
stomatitis 89, 120, 209
stroke see cerebrovascular accident 138–9
substance abuse 178–9
sugar
    consumption rate **15, 25, 26**
    reduction
        dietary care 24–7, 242
        in medicine 107–8, 141, 159–60, 184
surgery assistant training 81–2
Sydenham's chorea
swabs 113
swallow reflex see dysphagia
swallowing 217–18

T

tardive dyskinesia 176
tartar control 118
team dentistry 80–2
technician training 82
teeth
    development **44**
    effects of aging 58–9
temporomandibular joint
    arthritis 133
    pain 169
teratogens 108
terminal illness **222–3**
tetracycline 108
thalidomide 140
thalassaemias 188
therapist training 80–1
thrombocytopaenia 188
thrush see candidiasis
thymol glycerine 120
tongue-controlled switches 124

tooth care 24
    aids 68, **122–3**
    brush types **33**, 113, **114–17**, 123
    brushing 12, **49–51**, 81
    polishing 81
tooth loss
    distribution 17–18, 60–**1**
toothpastes 117–18
    pump-operated dispensers 123
toothpicks 117
Touch Tooth Kit 148
training
    nursing team 100–1
    oral assessment procedures 103–4
translucent teeth 135
transplants 185
trigeminal neuralgia 138
tuberculosis 189–90

U

ulcers
    elderly status 60–1
    osteoarthritis 133
    toxic reactions 108
unwaxed floss 115–16

V

varicella zoster 196–7
visits to dentist see appointments
visual impairment 148
vitamin deficiency 135
    B_{12} deficiency 187
    D absorption 135
von Willebrand's disease 188–9

W

ward-based oral care programme 101, 104
waxed floss 115–16
wood sticks 117
workplace
    oral health promotion 244–5

X

xerostomia 109, 121, 133, 160, 164–**6**, **191**
    208